The Definitive Guide

MEDICAL SCHOOL ADMISSION

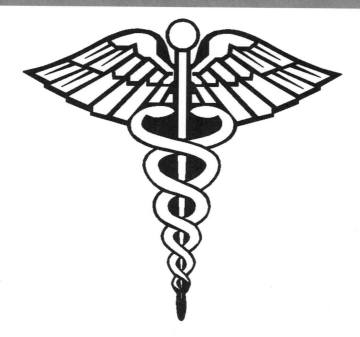

MARK A. GOLDSTEIN, M.D.
MYRNA CHANDLER GOLDSTEIN

Published by
Font & Center Press
P.O. Box 95
Weston, Massachusetts 02193

Book design by Becky Allen Mixter

Library of Congress Cataloging-in-Publication Data

Goldstein, Mark A. (Mark Allan), 1947–
    The definitive guide to medical school admission / Mark A.
    Goldstein, Myrna Chandler Goldstein.
        p.   cm.
    Includes bibliographical references and index.
    ISBN 1-883280-07-9
    1. Medical colleges—Entrance requirements.   2. Medical colleges—
Admission.   I. Goldstein, Myrna Chandler, 1948–   .   II. Title.
    [DNLM: 1. School Admission Criteria.   2. Education, Medical—
United States.   3. Schools, Mecical—United States—directories.
    4. Schools, Medical—Canada—directories.   W 18 G624d 1995]
R735.G65   1996
610'.71'173—dc20
DNLM/DLC
for Library of Congress   95-51107
                                                                      CIP

First Printing 1996
Printed in the United States of America

1 2 3 4 5 6 7 8 9 10

For Brett and Samantha

with love,

Mom and Dad

ACKNOWLEDGMENTS

I am most grateful to my spouse and co-author, Myrna Chandler Goldstein, for her efforts in reviewing my dictations and transposing the material into readable information. Her ability to create understandable, logical, and clearly written prose from my often rambling discourses is very much acknowledged. Her great patience and perseverance in working with me will be forever appreciated.

It is through the many meetings and countless questions from my advisees over the past years that I have attained and developed the information and format for this book. I am especially grateful to Monique Lawrence for her critical reading of the manuscript.

I appreciate the encouragement and suggestions from my physician colleagues, including Drs. Walter Rymzo, Chris Kryder, and Peter Reich.

There are several individuals who profoundly influenced me during my career. Mr. Allan Harrison, my high school biology teacher at the Walter Johnson High School in Rockville, Maryland, inspired me to pursue a medical career. Drs. Martin Myers at the Johns Hopkins Hospital, Nicola Tauraso at the N.I.H., Joseph Bellanti at Georgetown, and the late Nathan Talbot at the Massachusetts General Hospital all served as pediatrician role models. Dr. John Moses at M.I.T. could be best described as a doctor's doctor. I am especially grateful to Dr. Robert Masland of the Boston Children's Hospital, who to this day continues to be a model Adolescent Medicine physician.

My late uncle Albert Goldstein from Baltimore, a pioneer in the field of urology, a great clinician and surgeon, will always serve as my ideal physician.

M.A.G.

TABLE OF CONTENTS

LIST OF TABLES

INTRODUCTION

In the late 1960s, when I was an undergraduate at a state university, I knew that I wanted to attend medical school. In fact, pursuing a career in medicine had been my goal since early childhood. While I was aware of the basic courses required for medical school admission, I met only once with the premedical advisor. And that was probably just as well. He was an unfriendly man with a somewhat hostile manner. Rather than serving as a valued guide, his actions and demeanor more closely resembled those of an adversary. He provided no guidance. He never offered assistance with my applications, and he refused to let me view my letters of recommendation. My requests for preinterview coaching were denied. I remember quietly vowing that someday I would do something to correct the situation.

In spite of the odds, I was accepted to several medical schools and decided to attend Georgetown University School of Medicine. I graduated with the class of 1972.

Not everyone was so fortunate. Several of my friends, who also hoped for a career in medicine, were refused admission. Most attended graduate school in a related field. Others pursued completely different careers. Some still occasionally allude to their unfulfilled aspirations and wonder if they could have done something to change the course of events.

Although admission to medical school was competitive for my generation, today the odds are even more challenging. Simply put, more people are vying for the same number of openings.

For large numbers of people a career in medicine has enormous appeal. There is great excitement in the field, especially with regard to research, advances in therapy, basic sciences, genetics, and genetic engineering. And those who enter medicine may choose to practice in a multitude of ways. One may form or join a private practice;

teach in an academic setting; conduct basic or clinical research; serve as a dean or administrator for a medical school, clinic, or hospital; or work for a health maintenance organization, pharmaceutical company, or government agency. The opportunities are limitless. It is not at all unusual for physicians to work in several areas at the same time or at varying points in their careers.

Many areas of the U.S. economy have experienced long periods of recession or stagnant economic growth. All too often, professionals have found themselves to be middle-aged and out of work, but medicine and medical care is a growth industry. Finding a position is not difficult for a good, highly-trained physician.

It is not surprising that individuals choose medicine since it has so much to offer. Regrettably, most colleges and universities have insufficient resources to meet the advising needs of their premedical students. And, so, the vast majority of them receive essentially no guidance.

To complicate the situation even further, there is no formula that will guarantee admission to medical school. While one might assume that it is best to major in biology, in reality, admission to medical school is highest among those who major in history! And top grades and scores do not automatically open that stubborn medical school door. I have seen students with very high grades and MCAT scores be denied admission. Similarly, other students, who superficially appeared far less qualified, have gained a coveted place. Medical schools have accepted students who wanted to become physicians since early childhood and students who graduated from college in another field and then returned to fulfill premedical requirements.

This book should be useful to all premedical students. In addition, it may serve as a planning guide for middle school and high school students who are contemplating a future in medicine. Finally, it may be a resource for advisors. When I first began advising premedical students 17 years ago, I would have appreciated a book to help me prepare for the countless unanticipated situations that lay ahead.

This guide will walk the student through the entire application process — to help the applicant successfully master the many obstacles that he or she will encounter. Whenever possible, I have tried to include actual anecdotal experiences. While there is no guarantee that any one applicant will be accepted to medical school, proper planning and the development of an appropriate strategy may significantly improve your ability to portray yourself as a successful candidate to an admissions committee.

Best of luck for a future in medicine. Though the work may be hard and the hours long, I am still forever thankful that I have been able to pursue an exciting career that includes caring for children and adolescents, teaching medical students, interns, residents, and fellows; consulting; and advising premedical students. Every day when I wake up I am once again energized, knowing that the work that I do truly makes a difference.

Chapter One
. . . .

PREMEDICAL PREPARATION

Not all students wait until college to begin planning for medical school. Some know at a very young age — often in elementary or middle school — that they would like a career in medicine. And, so, these young people begin selecting specific courses and volunteering for certain programs that will stimulate and enhance this career goal.

I was such a kid. As a skinny eight-year-old, I was mesmerized by the workings of the human body and intrigued by all living things. Much to the chagrin of my mother, I collected every local animal including turtles, fish, birds, mice, rats, toads, frogs, hamsters, guinea pigs, dogs, and cats. After years of pleading for a chemistry set, I was overjoyed to receive one for my thirteenth birthday. Then, to the horror of my parents, I began formulating noxious and explosive compounds.

Doctors are people who prescribe medicine, of which they know little, to cure diseases, of which they know less, in human beings, of which they know nothing.

Voltaire

In my junior year of high school, my father died, and my mother was forced to scratch out a marginal income as a single-parent. Though family finances had always been tight, after the death of my father, it became necessary for me to devote most of my after-school and weekend hours to a host of different minimum wage jobs. I worried that I would be unable to realize my dream of a career in medicine.

Fortunately, we lived in Bethesda, Maryland, not far from the National Institutes of Health (NIH), and I entered a competition for a NIH research fellowship. Selection to one of the few slots enabled me spend the summer before my senior year totally immersed in research. I earned money for college while pursuing work that I loved. My life was turning around. I could not have been happier.

With top grades, very good scores on the college entrance examinations, that excellent NIH summer research opportunity, several science achievement awards, and countless hours of work, I should have been directed to apply to competitive colleges. Instead, like many other students with limited financial resources, I was told to attend our state university, a school with a policy of open admissions. There the yearly tuition would be only a few hundred dollars. It was not until several years later that I learned I was eligible to receive thousands of dollars in financial aid. Such assistance would have enabled me to attend a competitive college.

Don't repeat my mistake. There is absolutely no question that excelling at a strong, competitive college with an excellent premedical curriculum helps to open the doors to medical school. Table 1-1 indicates those colleges reporting 10 percent or more of their graduates and alumni attending medical school.

Strive to attend a highly competitive college. It is better to be a very good student in a highly competitive setting than an outstanding student in a noncompetitive environment. Although I was a top student at the state university, I would have been a better overall

---

Table 1-1

Schools Reporting 10 Percent or More of Graduates and Alumni Attending Medical School

Brandeis
Brown
Columbia
Davidson
Duke
Emory
Harvard
Johns Hopkins
MIT
NYU
Pomona
Stanford
Tufts
Washington University

Source: The College Handbook 1995.

premedical candidate had I been counseled to pursue a different course. The old saying is still appropriate. "Surrounding yourself with dwarfs will not make you a giant."

Which Courses are Required for Admission to Medical School?

Most medical schools require one year of biology, one year of inorganic or general chemistry, one year of organic chemistry, one year of physics, and one year of English. Some schools want a year of mathematics. According to the Association of American Medical Colleges (AAMC), 19 schools require calculus. Of course, these are the minimum course requirements. Extra courses in chemistry are useful if they do not duplicate medical school course work. Vertebrate embryology and genetics may also be desirable.

Nevertheless, it is equally important to enroll in classes that extend your intellectual breath. Choosing "gut" courses which will earn "A" grades and bolster your grade point average is unwise and inappropriate. Medical school admission committees are well aware of these offerings at various colleges. Consider your undergraduate years as an opportunity to broaden your intellect. If you do attend medical school, you will have little time for such pursuits.

Several years ago, Una K. Creditor and Morton C. Creditor, M.D., a Staff Associate and Interim Executive Dean at the University of Illinois College of Medicine, Chicago, compared the curriculum selections of premedical students to those of other students in the sciences and liberal arts. Although there were some weaknesses to their research design, the Creditors' found that premedical students enrolled in more science courses than other science and nonscience majors. And, when electing nonscience alternatives, they favored those in which they were likely to merit higher grades. Among the top 50 courses chosen by premedical students, there were very few nonscience subjects. When a nonscience class was picked, it was generally entry level. Rather than attempting to pursue a balanced undergraduate education, Creditor and Creditor found that premedical students chose courses in which high grades were virtually guaranteed.

Remember, the admissions committees are aware of this practice. You do not stand out from the crowd if you act like every other premedical student.

Some students believe that if they take more undergraduate science courses they will be better prepared for the rigorous medical school curriculum. To determine if that assumption had any basis in fact, David P. Yens, Ph.D., the Assistant Dean for Academic Affairs and Assistant Professor in the Department of Medical Education at Mt. Sinai School of Medicine, and Barry Stimmel, M.D., Dean for Academic Affairs, Admissions, and Student Affairs and Associate Professor, Department of Medicine, Mt. Sinai School of Medicine, studied the performance of four categories of undergraduate majors.

Yens and Stimmel examined nine classes of medical students at Mt. Sinai School of Medicine. Each student's premedical major was classified into one of four areas: traditional science, science using the scientific method, business, arts and humanities, or a health-related nonscience major. Criteria used to judge the students' performance included the undergraduate grade point average (GPA), Medical College Admission Test (MCAT) scores, course grades in medical school, and the result of the National Board of Medical Examiners testing.

While the authors found little variability in performance between the different majors, they noted that those students majoring in nonscience subjects seemed to do better in behavioral science and psychiatry. This study supports the contention that nonscience majors do as well as science majors in medical school.

Analogous findings were obtained by Judith Anderson Koenig, M.A., a Research Associate, Section for the Medical College Admission Test, at the AAMC, when she compared the performance of medical students who had a broad-based premedical education to those who had focused on premedical preparation. Broad-based preparation was defined as majoring in a nonscience discipline and participating in a wide variety of extracurricular activities, especially those unrelated to science or medicine such as athletics, journalism, or fine arts. Students focusing on science majored in the physical or biological sciences and had minimal course work in nonscience areas. Their extracurricular activities were related to science or medicine.

The study found differences in performance on the National Board of Medical Examiners Test Part I. Science-focused students scored higher on several science-oriented tests including biochemistry and physiology, while broad-based trained students scored higher on behavioral science tests. However, on Part II of the National Boards, which is usually administered in the senior year of medical school, the mean performance of both groups was similar. As a result, the study suggests that broad-based undergraduate preparation will not negatively affect the performance of students in medical school.

It has often been said that premedical students suffer from terminal cases of "premedical syndrome." They are excessively goal-oriented, compulsively over-achieving, obsessively concerned with grades, and ridiculously overspecialized. Studies, such as one conducted by Robert H. Sade, M.D., Professor of Cardiothoracic Surgery and Assistant Dean for Admissions at the Medical University of South Carolina, *et. al.*, have found that in comparison with their nonpremedical counterparts, premedical students do display many of the "premedical syndrome" characteristics. Still, these same students were also found to be self-disciplined, highly motivated, and proud of their career choice.

Although academic achievement is an important component in the medical school admissions decision, a premedical student should make every effort to counter the "premedical syndrome" image. It is never desirable to be too narrow, too competitive, or too cynical. And, as we shall see, you will improve your standing as a candidate and a future physician if you strive to become a more compassionate, well-rounded human being.

According to William C. McGaghie, Ph.D., Professor in the Office of Educational Development, University of North Carolina School of Medicine, admissions committees look for applicants with a "breadth of knowledge" rather than narrow specialization. A student who has amassed many science credits while essentially ignoring all other subjects and activities is seriously compromising his or her chances for admission. A broad "breadth of knowledge" will enhance a physician's daily practice of medicine and will facilitate interactions with patients, family members, and other members of the medical community. In a separate paper, McGaghie said that data collected by the AAMC showed that a "C plus" college GPA and an average MCAT score were usually sufficient to ensure orderly progress through medical school. McGaghie found that higher medical aptitude only translated into slight improvement in medical school achievement. As a result, McGaghie argues that medical school candidates should be selected for "nonacademic" factors. Graduation rates would not be affected, he says, by students who had a minimal college GPA and an average MCAT score. But, it is obvious from data, that this practice is not being followed by the vast majority of medical colleges.

Rudolph H. Weingartner, Dean of the College of Arts and Sciences, Northwestern University, goes even further. He strongly discourages selecting a premedical major and contends that medical schools should insist that every applicant give evidence of a broad undergraduate education. This may be accomplished in one of two ways. Either avoid majoring in biology, biochemistry, or chemistry or enroll in a number of introductory and advanced courses in the humanities and social sciences. Weingartner insists that all medical students earn a bachelor's degree. And while he admits that good grades are important, he thinks that it is absurd to maintain that a student with a 3.76 GPA is a better candidate than one with a GPA of 3.65.

David Sarnoff, the broadcasting pioneer who established the first radio network, NBC, once noted, "Competition brings out the best in products and the worst in people." And the insightful Albert Einstein cautioned, "Try not to become a man of success but rather a man of value."

Foreign Language

Foreign language is another important issue. I studied Latin in high school and French in college. If I could do it over, I would choose Latin and Spanish. The derivatives I learned in Latin proved useful in anatomy. And, several years later, Spanish would have been invaluable when I spent one year as a Public Health Service physician in a Spanish-speaking community in New Mexico. In my current practice of medicine in Boston and Cambridge, a familiarity with Spanish would also be advantageous. Spanish is becoming increasingly important in the practice of medicine. Fluency in Russian or Asian languages may also be helpful since there are increasing numbers of Russian and Asian immigrants.

What is the Best Major?

While this may shatter numerous myths, it is essential to mention that **there is no ideal premedical major**. At the same time, there is no major that should, at all costs, be avoided.

Although significant numbers of premedical students are biology or chemistry majors, there are some schools that make a point of selecting students who major in nonscience areas. I do not believe that there is any advantage to majoring in science. In fact, at certain schools, science majors have a distinct disadvantage.

According to the AAMC, for applicants to the 1994–95 entering class to American medical schools, 45.7 percent of the students had majored in biological sciences and 17.1 percent had majored in the physical sciences. The remainder had majored in nonscience subjects, mixed disciplines, or entered medical school from other health professions. Further data from the AAMC indicates that 35.7 percent of the accepted students majored in biological science. In comparison, 42.1 percent of those majoring in the physical sciences were offered a space. At the same time, over 50 percent of the history majors were accepted. In the entering class for 1994–95, there were 581 applicants who majored in history. Of these, 301 were admitted. That is a 51.8 percent acceptance rate! History majors had the highest acceptance rate of all majors. On the other hand, the lowest acceptance rate was for individuals from other health professions including nursing, pharmacy, and medical technology. These data substantiate the fact that nonscience majors may have a strong application.

I advise you to major in a subject you truly enjoy. Since admission to medical school is never guaranteed, you may find that your life's work will ultimately be in that major. Select it carefully and with great thought.

Should you consider a double major? If you want a double major based on your intellectual interests, that's fine. Do not assume that it will, necessarily, strengthen your application. Admissions committees like to see quality work. You need only major in one area to do that. Though achieving a master's degree while still an undergraduate is commendable and may be helpful, it is certainly neither the norm nor the expectation. But I would caution against applying to medical school following the completion of only three years of college. Most medical schools require four years of college or an undergraduate degree. Medical schools look askance at applicants who want to shave one year off their premedical planning. It is well known that during that treasured senior year, you may enrich your background by selecting elective courses. Recently, I had an advisee who was able to graduate after only three years in college. Because the fourth year of undergraduate education would place a financial burden on his family, he decided to apply to medical school based on the three years. He was admitted to several. While his application would have been stronger if he had the fourth year, since he had the degree, I believe his decision was appropriate. However, in general, four years of college and an undergraduate degree are the expectation. And exceptions to the rule should be rare.

References — Chapter One

1. *The College Handbook 1995,* 32nd edition, College Entrance Examination Board, 1994.
2. *Medical School Admission Requirements 1996–97,* Association of American Medical Colleges, 1995.
3. Creditor, U.K., Creditor, M.C., "Curriculum Choices of Premedical Students," *Journal of Medical Education,* 57:436–441, 1982.
4. Yens, D.P., Stimmel, B., "Science Verses Nonscience Undergraduate Studies for Medical School: A Study of Nine Classes," *Journal of Medical Education,* 57:429–435, 1982.
5. Koenig, J.A., "Comparison of Medical School Performances and Career Plans of Students with Broad and with Science-focused Premedical Preparation," *Academic Medicine,* 67:191–196, 1992.
6. Sade, R.M., Fleming, G.A., Ross, G.R., "A Survey on the 'Premedical Syndrome,'" *Journal of Medical Education,* 59:386–391, 1984.
7. McGaghie, W.C., "Qualitative Variables in Medical School Admission," *Academic Medicine,* 65:145–148, 1990.
8. McGaghie, W.C., "Perspectives on Medical School Admission," *Academic Medicine,* 65:136–139, 1990.
9. Weingartner, R.H., "Selecting for Medical School," *Journal of Medical Education,* 55:922–927, 1980.

Chapter Two

· · · · · · · ·

FACTORS INFLUENCING SELECTION

I would venture to guess that even before you opened this book you knew that applications to medical schools far exceeded the available spaces. That may well be one of the reasons that you decided to read what I have to say.

Few would disagree that gaining admission to medical schools is no easy feat. In recent years, with more students applying for the same number of slots, the intense competition has only escalated. Every year the medical schools reject far more students than they accept. And, faced with so many qualified candidates, it is likely that admissions committees sometimes bypass students who might well have become excellent physicians.

There is no such

· · · · · · · · · · · · · · · ·

thing as a free lunch

Milton Friedman

As in many other areas of life, knowledge is vital. You must take the time to learn about the admissions process and what will make you shine before the discerning eyes and ears of the members of the admissions committees.

So, what are the selection factors used by admissions committees? I believe that there are several general sets of criteria which I have classified into four categories: quantitative, qualitative, demographic, and "soft."

Quantitative Criteria

The quantitative criteria may be subdivided into the applicant's grade point average (GPA), the applicant's science GPA, the result of the applicant's Medical College Admission Test (MCAT), and the selectivity of the college attended by the applicant.

Of all the criteria, the GPA is probably the most widely used. While not all medical schools report GPA statistics, of those medical schools that provide such data to the Association of American Medical Colleges (AAMC), the majority indicate that, on a 4.0 scale, for the school year 1993–94 their first year students had earned an undergraduate mean GPA between 3.3 and 3.7, with many hovering between 3.4 and 3.5. For the Harvard Medical School class of 1999, the mean grade point average for the incoming class was close to 3.75 out of 4.00 according to *Focus*, a publication of the Harvard Medical, Dental, and School of Public Health.

Although the GPA is an extremely important quantitative measure, it is very far from an absolute guarantee of admission or rejection. I have had advisees with high GPAs who have assumed that they would automatically be granted admission. They were wrong. On the other hand, I have had advisees with GPAs of 2.8 who were accepted. Nevertheless, assuming other factors are equal, as your GPA rises, so do your chances for admission.

It is very important to remember that GPAs are not earned in a vacuum. Members of admissions committees know that it is much harder to maintain a high GPA at a competitive college. And GPAs will be evaluated accordingly.

More than a decade ago, Randolph E. Sarnacki, Ph.D., the Assistant Director of Educational Research and Evaluation and an Assistant Professor of Social and Preventive Medicine at the State University of New York at Buffalo School of Medicine, examined the relative usefulness of the GPA in distinguishing between applicants to medical school and in predicting the performance of applicants accepted to medical school. Students from two graduating classes of the State University of New York at Buffalo Medical School were evaluated on several groups of measurements. The first group included scores on the science subtest of the MCAT, undergraduate science GPAs, and undergraduate GPAs. The second group consisted of performance in basic science during the first two years of medical school. And the third group reflected the results of Part I and Part II examinations of the National Board of Medical Examiners. The selectivity of undergraduate colleges was determined by Barron's College Admission Selector. The Barron's index uses freshman class mean SAT scores, the percentage of students scoring above 500, 600, and 700 on sections of the SAT, the grade average or rank from high school, and the proportion of applicants offered admission by the college.

Sarnacki's investigation found that students from the "most competitive" colleges had total GPAs and mean-entering-science GPAs that were lower than students from "competitive" colleges. While that in itself would tend to support the college weighting theory, there is even more evidence. For though the GPAs varied according to the competitive levels of the colleges, the science subtest of the MCAT — an equal-opportunity tester — showed far less variability. Once in medical school, the students displayed no significant differences in GPAs or in results of the National Board of Medical Examiners Examinations. Weighting undergraduate GPAs levels the playing field and helps to select students who will perform equally well in medical school.

After studying institutional selectivity as a predictor of success in medical school, Terry T. Clapp, Ed.D., Assistant Professor and Coordinator, Allied Health Science Education, Northern Arizona University, and John C. Reid, Ph.D., Professor of Education and Evaluation Specialist, Educational Resources Group, University of Missouri–Columbia Medical Center, found that the GPA, adjusted by the selectivity of the institution, is far more important than overall GPA. For example, let's say you have earned a GPA of 3.9 at a non-competitive college. Since you just read that most medical schools require a GPA between 3.3 and 3.7, you might be tempted to assume that your chances for admission are excellent. *Wrong!* Similarly, if you have a far lower GPA at the most competitive school — let's say a 2.7 — you might conclude that it would be a waste of time, effort, and money to even consider applying. *Wrong again!*

> *Nothing ever comes to one that is worth having except as a result of hard work.*
>
> **Booker T. Washington**

Obviously, the admissions committees are interested in your science GPA. It reflects your performance in courses that are basic to medical school training — biology, general chemistry, organic chemistry, and physics. However, I do not believe that it is absolutely imperative that you earn an "A" in any one course. When I was a premedical undergraduate, everyone felt that medical schools required an "A" in organic chemistry. Well, I didn't earn an "A." For me, organic chemistry was extraordinarily difficult. Frankly, I considered myself fortunate to earn "A"s and "B"s. While an "A" in organic chemistry is not a necessity, a truly bad grade, such as a "D", will certainly hurt you. And it might indicate that you should consider another career choice rather than medical school.

Once I had an advisee who earned a "D" in organic chemistry. His choice was clear. He could apply to medical school and be fairly certain of rejection. Or, he could repeat the course. At my suggestion, he repeated the course and earned an "A". Eventually, he was accepted to medical school. Though the "D" still appeared on his transcript, as his premedical advisor, I was able to include a modifier explaining that he had been ill that term. The "A" that was later earned reflected his true ability to complete the course work.

Work as hard as you possibly can in all of your premedical courses. While a premedical student who majors in history will present a very different transcript than one who majors in Spanish, they both will have completed similar premedical requirements. And those grades carry a significant weight.

The MCAT, which will be discussed in greater detail in Chapter Five, is also very important. All applicants are required to take the MCAT, and its scores are standardized. As a result, it is the one measure that equally evaluates science, math, verbal reasoning, and writing ability. Of course, we all know that some people are better test takers than others and that people have good days and days that are not so great. And, no one would deny that one day's performance is less important than work completed during three years of college. Nevertheless, do not underestimate the value of this test or the role that it plays in the admissions process. The average MCAT subtest score for the Harvard Medical School class of 1999 was approximately 11 according to the article in *Focus.*

Frances R. Hall, Ed.M., Assistant Dean for Admission and Financial Aid, Dartmouth Medical School, and Beth A. Bailey, M.A., Assistant Director of Admissions, University of Virginia School of Medicine, correlated students' undergraduate science GPAs, the MCAT scores, and the selectivity of the colleges with first year performance at Dartmouth Medical School. For their study they reviewed five different classes — 420 students entering Dartmouth Medical School from 1982 to 1986. Collected data included undergraduate science, nonscience, and total GPAs, MCAT scores, selectivity of undergraduate institutions, grades earned in each first year medical school course, and the total first year GPA.

Using the mean SAT for admission, Hall and Bailey classified the students' undergraduate schools into different groups — low selectivity, intermediate selectivity, and high selectivity. The five year mean GPA in science from students at low selectivity schools was 3.43. That stands in contrast to a mean GPA of 3.37 from students at intermediate selectivity schools or 3.15 from students at high selectivity schools. Entering students showed no significant difference in MCAT scores. First-year medical school GPAs were also very similar.

Again, it is evident that admissions committees weigh the academic caliber of undergraduate colleges. In this particular case, they were weighed so well that the students' performance was consistent despite the selectivity rating of his or her college.

A few years ago, Karen J. Mitchell, Assistant Vice President for Educational Research and Director MCAT Program at the AAMC, reviewed the traditional predictors of performance in medical school. To evaluate undergraduate achievement, she examined undergraduate grades, college selectivity, transcript data, and MCAT performance. Medical school performance was determined by basic sciences grades, clinical sciences grades, scores on the National Board of Medical Examiners Examinations Part I, II, and III, and information on students experiencing academic difficulty.

Mitchell reaffirmed the value of the traditional academic predictors of performance in medical school. In other words, if you did well as an undergraduate and did well on the MCAT, you will probably do well in medical school. Acknowledging the significance of these indicators, Mitchell also advises admissions committees to consider nonacademic information and material gleaned from the interview. I agree. The brightest student from the most selective college may not have the qualitative characteristics so important for a future physician.

Qualitative Characteristics

Though admissions committee members may find it hard to measure qualitative characteristics, they are still an integral part of the selection process. And as you prepare to present yourselves to schools, you should keep them at the forefront of your thoughts.

Integrity

In my opinion, the most meaningful qualitative characteristic is integrity. Unfortunately, it is also the most difficult for an admissions committee to ascertain or for an applicant to prove. All of us want our physicians to be honest. In recent years, there have been too many examples of dishonest research, medical insurance fraud, and the overprescription of controlled drugs for unsound medical reasons.

So how does one demonstrate integrity? For most applicants, letters of reference from the applicant's premedical advisor and respected members of the university community will serve as the ideal vehicle for documenting integrity. Such letters should be written by people who know the applicant very well, and they should include personal anecdotes. The candidate may also have opportunities during the interview or through the personal statement to demonstrate integrity.

Leadership

A second important characteristic is leadership. Why leadership? Physicians are generally expected to assume leadership roles in their local communities and in the larger society. Moreover, medical training, especially residency, requires the ability to lead and to direct others. How does one prove leadership ability? Become a member of the student government, president of your social or religious organization or fraternity, quarterback of the football team, or crew coxswain. If you submit an application devoid of leadership ability, then you may well find yourself relegated to the bottom of the applicant pile.

Motivation

Motivation is another key qualitative characteristic. It is to your advantage to present yourself as a high energy applicant who is motivated to perform well in college and in extracurricular activities. Taking the more demanding courses while continuing involvement in extracurricular activities and possibly research or volunteer work, help demonstrate a motivated student.

Curiosity

Then there is curiosity. Though it is not clear if medical schools actually seek students who are curious, it is certainly true that every physician should be a naturally inquisitive individual who repeatedly looks beyond the easiest or most obvious answer or solution. It is always refreshing to see a curious medical student make the time to research clinical problems he or she observes on a clinical rotation. That extra measure of curiosity helps the student to gain a greater depth of clinical knowledge. As an undergraduate, one way to show curiosity would be to participate in research projects in medicine, a medically related field, engineering, mathematics, humanities, or any other field.

Imagination

Still another important characteristic is imagination. Imaginative researchers don't just ask questions. They see solutions and answers — sometimes very unusual ones — that occasionally work. Let's consider, for example, the researchers who were looking for a way to prevent Hepatitis B. Previously, the only vaccine used against this virulent virus was made from pooled human sera. Regrettably, this caused negative reactions in people. Imaginative researchers used recombinant technology to develop a vaccine that produces immunity to Hepatitis B while remaining free from any infectious particles and human sera. So now that one group of researchers has used imagination to create this vaccine, another group, practicing physicians, must draw on their own imagination to encourage groups such as adolescents to receive the vaccinations. One way might be to organize an art contest where contestants create art promoting increased use of this vaccine.

Imagination is the highest kite one can fly.

Lauren Bacall

It is now up to you to draw on your own curiosity and imagination to prove to the members of an admissions committee that you do indeed have these valuable characteristics. It's not easy. But no one ever said that the road to medical school would be smoothly paved.

Personality

Without a doubt, all of us would like our physicians to be friendly, compassionate, and congenial human beings. But we all know that personalities vary among all people, including physicians. During your interview(s), feel free to be yourself. But try not to be too friendly or too formal. If you tend to be very outgoing, try mixing in a drop of reserve. If you tend to be extremely withdrawn, try to be more open. It is definitely unwise to be combative or overly anxious. If it is evident that you find the interview process too stressful, the interviewer might wonder how you would manage a trauma case in the emergency room or a heart attack in the intensive care unit. Consider yourself very fortunate if you and your interviewer are compatible.

Volunteer Service

For several reasons, I require that every one of my premedical advisees volunteer at a hospital. First, I think that it is imperative that a premedical student be exposed to a hospital environment where he or she plans to spend many months of training and countless years of a future career. Sometimes, students who volunteer realize that they are uncomfortable in the hospital setting and decide not to pursue a career in medicine. Clearly, it is better to make that decision before entering medical school.

Altruism

Working as a physician also requires a certain degree of altruism. Volunteering in a hospital — a form of altruism or caring for others — is an ideal means to serve others while determining if medicine is your true calling. It should also be noted that some medical school admissions committees consider public service to be an important selection criterion.

Demographic Characteristics

Demographic characteristics include an applicant's state of residence, gender, age, nationality, and race. All of these factors may be used to some degree by admissions committees.

There is no question that the state of residence is important to state medical schools. A number of these admit few nonresident applicants. While the other factors — gender, age, nationality, and race — are considered in the admissions process, members of admissions committees only acknowledge an effort "to balance" the classes. To indicate that they attempt to admit a specific number of students of either gender might leave them legally liable.

According to George Nowacek, Ph.D., Director of the Office of Medical Education and Associate Professor of Medical Education at the University of Virginia School of Medicine, and Larry Sachs, Ph.D., Associate Director of the School of Allied Medical Professions at Ohio State University, the federal law is very clear. One may not use gender in screening applicants or in admissions decisions.

Research suggests that significant numbers of students who were raised in rural settings return to practice in a rural community. As a result, some medical schools, particularly state medical schools hoping to graduate students who will practice primary medicine in rural communities, may use a student's hometown as criterion for admission.

Race is a consideration. Often, medical schools will give data on the number of students who have been accepted under affirmative action programs.

"Soft" Criteria

While less important than some other factors, my final category of "soft" criteria should be reviewed by those applying to medical school. You never can tell. It might just be one minor consideration that could make the difference in your application.

Harrison G. Gough, Ph.D., Professor of Psychology at the University of California and Director of the Institute of Personality Assessment and Research, and Wallace B. Hall, Ph.D., Associate Research Psychologist at the Institute, compared medical students at the University of California, San Francisco, School of Medicine, who were from medical and nonmedical families. Of the 1,195 students from 11 classes, 162 were from medical and 1,033 were from nonmedical families. Their findings are interesting. Students who had fathers or mothers who were physicians had similar premedical achievement and MCAT scores to students in the larger group. However, they were slightly younger and generally attended more prestigious undergraduate colleges. Once in medical school, both groups performed equally well. Nevertheless, they did differ in residency selections. The students who had medical parents tended to specialize in ophthalmology (eyes), otorhinolaryngology (ears, nose, and throat), dermatology, or surgery. They were less likely to pick pediatrics, psychiatry, or obstetrics/gynecology. In all probability, for the vast majority of applicants, having a parent who is a physician has a minimal effect on the selection process. For a small minority, who may apply to the medical school attended by a parent, it could have some small impact.

Letters of reference from medical school faculty members, particularly faculty at the schools you would most wish to attend, may be useful. You could work with a medical school professor during a summer research opportunity. Each year, I have been able to connect one of my advisees or another premedical student to a research opportunity at a Harvard teaching hospital. And it is not at all far fetched to say that admissions committee members may give more weight to letters written by their own faculty members.

Consider it a true gift if admissions committee members are personally acquainted with those faculty members.

If you are an undergraduate within a university system that has its own medical school, you may have a slight advantage over students applying from other colleges and universities. And, if your relatives — particularly parents, grandparents, or siblings — attended medical schools, then you should strongly consider applying to those schools as well. In such a competitive market, even the smallest soft criterion could give you that extra edge.

Finally, you should review the admissions information in the catalogue of each medical school you are considering. Occasionally, you will find medical schools with unique or particular selection factors. The following details have been gathered from the Infact Medical School Information System which has the recent catalogue of each American and Canadian medical school on microfiche.

Columbia

The Committee places great importance on the fact that the students have learned to think for themselves, to explore, to work hard under their own initiative, to consider alternatives and make decisions, and to develop a desire for a continuous program of self-education. In the selection of the students, preference is given to those who, in the opinion of the Committee on Admissions, have shown high achievement in their college education, a mature sense of values, sound motivation, qualities of leadership, and ability to assume responsibility, and to those who have already given evidence that they are qualified to complete all requirements of our curriculum and to graduate as ethical, compassionate, and competent physicians.

Cornell

In addition to objective criteria . . . evaluation of applicants also involved subjective judgments including an assessment of student motivation, maturity, stability, and other factors deemed by the faculty to be essential for the education of an effective and competent physician. . . . Well-motivated students from particularly adverse economic or social backgrounds who have the substandard educational opportunities are seriously considered.

Duke

Good study habits, intelligence, character, and integrity are essential qualifications for admission. Beyond this, premedical students should strive for an education that develops abilities to observe critically, think analytically, and work independently. Though a knowledge of basic scientific principles should be secured, the competence with which premedical students conduct their undergraduate careers is of more importance than the specific subjects which they study.

Georgetown
Students are selected on the basis of academic achievement, character, maturity, and motivation.

Howard
Candidates for admission and alternates are from those applicants who have competitive academic credentials, desirable personal and social traits, and who are most likely to practice in communities or facilities needing physician services.

University of Pennsylvania
The choice of students is made on the basis of the opinion of the Committee of Admissions regarding the applicant's character, ability, fitness to pursue the study of medicine, and promise for the future. This is determined by many including the academic standards of the college at which the applicant prepared, performance in academic courses, the record of activity in extracurricular college and community affairs, Medical College Admission Test scores, and information offered by the applicant's college faculty.

Rochester
Success in medicine depends on many attributes. Scholastic accomplishment is only one. The Medical Admissions Committee gives careful consideration to many other factors, including integrity, judgment, maturity, general knowledge, and special aptitudes.

Stanford
The School of Medicine is interested in candidates who have a strong humanitarian commitment and who show evidence of originality, creativity, and a capacity for independent, critical thinking. Enthusiasm for the basic sciences and outstanding accomplishment in those areas are prerequisites for admission to the school, but the Committee on Admissions also looks for evidence of breadth of education and/or experience in the humanities and social sciences.

UCLA
Preference is given to students who, in the opinion of the Admissions Committee, present evidence of broad training and high achievement in college, an interest in biomedical research, a capacity

to develop mature interpersonal relationships, and the traits of personality and character which mark the competent, conscientious, and compassionate physician.

Washington University

Evidence of superior intellectual ability and scholastic achievement. . . . Evidence of character, a caring and compassionate attitude, scientific and humanitarian interests, and motivation suitable for a career in medicine.

Yale

The Committee on Admissions in general seeks to admit students who seem best suited for the educational programs and aims of the School. In particular, it looks for intelligent, mature, and highly motivated students who show the greatest promise for becoming leaders and contributors in medicine. The Committee on Admissions also considers very carefully personal qualities necessary for the successful student and practice of medicine. These include integrity, common sense, personal stability, dedication to the ideal of service, and the ability to inspire and maintain confidence.

References — Chapter Two

1. *Medical School Admission Requirements 1996–97,* Association of American Medical Colleges, 1995.
2. Sauber, C., "Doctor Still Has an Allure," *Focus,* September 5, 1995.
3. Sarnacki, R.E., "The Predictive Value of the Premedical Grade-Point Average," *Journal of Medical Education,* 57:163–169, 1982.
4. Clapp, T.T., Reid, J.C., "Institutional Selectivity as a Predictor of Applicant Selection and Success in Medial School," *Journal of Medical Education,* 51:850–852, 1976.
5. Hall, F.R., Bailey, B.A., "Correlating Students' Undergraduate Science GPAs, Their MCAT Scores, and the Academic Caliber of Their Undergraduate Colleges With Their First-Year Academic Performances Across Five Classes at Dartmouth Medical School," *Academic Medicine,* 67:121–123, 1992.
6. Mitchell, K.J., "Traditional Predictors of Performance in Medical School," *Academic Medicine,* 65:149–158, 1990.
7. Nowacek, G., Sachs, L., "Demographic Variables in Medical School Admission," *Academic Medicine,* 65:140–144, 1990.
8. Gough, H.G., Hall, W.B., "A Comparison of Medical Students From Medical and Nonmedical Families," *Journal of Medical Education,* 52:541–546, 1977.
9. Infact Medical School Information System. Dataflow Systems, Inc., Bethesda, Maryland.

Chapter Three

PREMEDICAL ADVISING

While the programs vary from school to school, just about all universities and colleges have members of the faculty and staff who serve as premedical advisors. Often, these are people with an interest in biology, chemistry, or physics.

Many colleges and universities go a step further — they have formed premedical councils. Members of these councils are responsible for advising premedical students and writing letters of recommendation. In general, these councils are part of a pre-professional office which is directed by a member of the faculty or staff. Such offices have reference libraries and personnel to answer questions and coordinate the mailing of letters of recommendation. In colleges and universities where the premedical population is considerable — sometimes as high as 25 percent of the student body — this office may be a very busy place.

Better ask twice than

lose your way once.

Danish Poverb

The premedical advisor serves a number of functions. At the minimum, he or she is a source for information on application dates, course and testing requirements, and individual medical schools. If the advisor is more experienced and has some extra time, then he or she may offer additional assistance and a wealth of information to the premedical student.

In a small minority of schools, such as the Massachusetts Institute of Technology (MIT), many of the premedical advisors are also physicians. At MIT, this is a result of a rather unusual situation. Unlike most colleges and universities, MIT has its own full-service medical department that provides medical services to the entire MIT community. In addition, some physicians are faculty at the Harvard-MIT Division of Health Sciences and Technology. Thus, MIT is blessed with an abundance of physicians who devote a small but significant portion of their time to premedical advising. I am one of this group.

Over my years of advising, I have found that a specific schedule of meetings appears to best serve the needs of my premedical advisees and provide opportunities for students to have their advising questions answered. Ideally, I first meet a premedical advisee in the middle of sophomore year for about 30 minutes. Then, in the junior year we meet twice — once in the fall and a second time in the spring. These early meetings enable me to better understand the individual student. I learn about future career goals and academic progress. I hear stories of triumph and frustration. And, over time, I am able to determine if the student has what it takes to make a committed and caring physician. In short, by the June prior to senior year, when the medical school application process gains momentum, I am well acquainted with the student. At the June meeting we together develop a list of at least 15 medical schools to which the student will apply. In July, we review the application personal statement and curriculum vitae. Our final meeting, which is held in the fall before the interview process has begun, is a mock application interview. I try to help the student understand effective interviewing strategies. (The interview will be discussed in more detail in Chapter Seven: The Interview.)

If a student has been accepted to several medical schools or if a student has not been admitted to any medical school, there is frequently a final meeting to discuss available options. When a student is placed on the waiting list of a school he or she would like to attend, I am able to contact the school by letter and/or telephone. After being contacted directly by a premedical advisor, some schools will place students at the top of the waiting list.

As you can see, premedical advising requires a substantial time commitment, especially when one is advising several students. I have found, however, that it is well worth the effort. And it is best not to rush the process. When steps have been bypassed, I have been of less assistance as an advisor, and I certainly have less material to include in the letter of recommendation. During the two years in which I advise each student, a seemingly endless number of questions are raised. Students ask about the medical school admission process, course work, and how to respond when one's academic status changes. For example, when a premedical student fails a course or receives a "D," there is a need for appropriate counseling and a proactive reaction. Also, there are specific ways to respond when I learn that a student has received a low score on the MCAT. Those will be discussed in detail later in the book.

A number of my advisees have asked if switching from engineering to premedicine late in the college career hurts their chances for admission to medical school. Clearly, these applicants need to be able to justify their switch either in the personal statement or during the interview. I am happy to say that most of my "late switches" have been admitted to medical school.

The Letter of Recommendation

Many people consider the recommendation written by the premedical advisor to be the most important letter in the student's portfolio. When writing this letter, utmost care must be taken to give an accurate description of the student's accomplishments and to portray qualities and characteristics not readily identified in the application. In some cases, this recommendation should offer an explanation for a problem in the student's application.

My letters of recommendation are not written in a vacuum. During the meetings with advisees, I learn a great deal. I also compile folders on each student. Ideally, the folder contains my notes on the individual student, an up-to-date curriculum vitae, letters of recommendation from three or four college faculty and/or staff, MCAT scores, a transcript, and a copy of the AMCAS personal statement. By the time I write the recommendation, I have a wealth of information at my fingertips.

The letter of recommendation should not be written in a dispassionate or semi-scientific style. In fact, the more narrative and personable the letter, the better it will describe the student. And the letter should not be more than one and one-half pages, single-spaced. The first and last paragraphs are the most important. People who read medical school applications often skim the body of the letter and read only the introduction and conclusion.

In every letter of recommendation, I try to answer the following questions:

1. Is this student intellectually capable to succeed in medical school?
2. How does this student rank when compared to my current and previous advisees?
3. Has the student excelled in any special way or been recognized by others for singular achievements?
4. Are there any problems that should be explained?

One year I had an advisee who was involved, with his mother, in a serious motor vehicle accident. Although he survived, his mother died. For a period of time, his grades suffered. It is imperative for an admissions committee to know this information.

As I write my letters, I am very careful to use the appropriate adjectives. Clearly, I am not able to write that every advisee is an outstanding candidate. Yes, some students are outstanding. But others are excellent, and others are good. Fair candidates should probably not apply.

It is very important for premedical advisors not to downplay the importance of this letter. The letter is crucial to the student's application, and it must be very carefully written. An incorrect adjective or innuendo could hurt the student's chances for admission. Take time with this letter. Be thoughtful. Incisive. Perceptive. Your words have power. And it is a power that must never be abused.

The following are examples of letters of recommendation. While the content is accurate, I have changed the names of people, departments, institutions, and some of the wording. In the first letter, I must account for the relatively low MCAT scores of an otherwise excellent candidate.

Jane Conway Doe
August 22, 1994

It is a distinct honor as her premedical advisor, to write this letter of recommendation on behalf of Jane Conway Doe who is applying for the medical school class entering September 1995. During our meetings over the past two years, I have been able to develop a picture of Ms. Doe which I shall present to you.

Ms. Doe came to MIT in 1991 having graduated in the top five percent of her high school class in Any Town, USA. She decided to major in chemistry with a minor in African-American studies and will graduate from MIT one term early in December 1994. Her academic achievements have been excellent in a difficult major. Ms. Doe's MCAT scores do not fairly portray her intellectual abilities. During her tenure at MIT, Ms. Doe has demonstrated great accomplishments in two areas: research and public service. On my encouragement, Ms. Doe applied for and was accepted into a research program at the XYZ Service of the Super Great Hospital, Harvard Medical School. Under the tutelage of Dr. ZZZ, Ms. Doe has undertaken a study of a very important disease related to the individual's fluid intake during hospitalization. She has continued this research for two years and received accolades from her mentor. In the area of public service, Ms. Doe was recently selected as one of three outstanding individuals (out of a pool of 250). This is quite a high honor that MIT bestows on a student. Ms. Doe has also volunteered for two years on the school-age childrens' floor of the Super Great Hospital.

Jane Conway Doe is an outstanding candidate for admission to medical school. If there is any weakness in her portfolio, it is the MCAT scores which do not truly account for her abilities. While coming from a nonphysician family, Ms. Doe has been motivated to enter medicine since early childhood. She has the ideal blend, in my view, of an aspiring future physician: outstanding intellect, strong commitment to public service, a curiosity and gift for research, and an impeccable integrity.

As a physician who not only advises premedical students, but also teaches medical students in all classes, I have a unique perspective. Ms. Doe fulfills all of the criteria I hope to observe in medical students. Clearly, she should be and will be admitted to medical school, and I predict she will be an outstanding physician in her chosen field. Since I am convinced she will be a success in medical school, I would enjoy being her pediatric attending physician.

This second letter was prepared for a naturalized citizen applying to an M.D./Ph.D. program.

Claude Bernard
August 3, 1995

Claude Bernard is one of the half dozen or so best premedical students that I have advised since 1979. Here is an individual with the intellect, scientific curiosity, flair with people, and communication skills who will be an outstanding medical student and physician.

After graduating as valedictorian of his high school in New York City, Mr. Bernard arrived at MIT in September 1992. He selected a challenging major — Biochemical Engineering — and has performed in an outstanding manner. Although his freshman grades are reported as pass, in fact, most, if not all of them, were "A" level. Professor XYZ felt he was one of the most talented students in his science laboratory class. His literature professor, AAAA RRRR said Claude was one of the very best students in his many years of teaching at MIT. Although his initial MCAT scores suffered because Mr. Bernard had a severe migraine headache on test day, in fact the repeat scores are outstanding.

In the laboratory Mr. Bernard has worked with Professor CBA on the mechanism of pathogensis of a very important brain disease. He has syntheized peptides from a critical region of the amyloid protein found in patients with this disease. It is my understanding that Mr. Bernard has worked extremely well in the lab with a sophistication not always found in doctoral students.

One could have the misconception that an MIT student at the top of his class with distinction in the laboratory could not also have excellent relationships with people. The reality is that Claude is committed to people. He works well with peers, professors, and patients. He is very much involved with our community, and he values public service.

As a writer for our student newspaper, *The Tech*, Mr. Bernard demonstrates his written skills. Several of his professors comment positively on his writing ability even though English is his second language. He is able to tutor and teach his peers with great competence.

As his premedical advisor, I have had the fortune to know Mr. Bernard during his entire MIT career. It was very clear to me from our first meeting in 1992, that he was an exceptional person. During these three years, he has demonstrated to me that he has the highest integrity, motivation, and honesty — characteristics which are so important for future physicians. It is also clear that he has the burning desire to enter the field of medicine. I note this charactertistic only occasionally in my advisees, but I cherish it when I find it.

One fortunate medical school will convince Mr. Bernard to attend. He is a very special person and I am sure he will become an outstanding physician who will be an asset to our profession. As one of my best advisees during my career, he has my highest recommendation for admission to the most competitive medical schools.

This recommendation was written for a truly outstanding student.

Clara Barton
September 8, 1992

It is a distinct honor and pleasure to write this letter of recommendation on behalf of Clara Barton who is applying for admission to the medical school class entering September 1993. As her premedical advisor, I have known Ms. Barton since early 1991.

Ms. Barton came to MIT with a very distinguished record from the Academic High School in Anywhere, USA. At MIT, she has continued an exemplary record in academics as well as extracurricular activities. Let me cite a few examples. Her almost perfect overall "A" average includes work in advanced and difficult academic subjects. She has performed in an exemplary manner in research laboratories at the Dana Farber Cancer Center, Stanford, University of California San Francisco, and MIT. Her classmates have elected her to important leadership positions including class officer for all four years and vice president of her sorority.

I asked Ms. Barton to help devise a seminar program for incoming freshman in the MIT class of 1996. With great enthusiasm she helped plan and then lead a very successful seminar. She is now writing an article on how to be successful at MIT which will be published this November in a newsletter I edit. Ms. Barton has great sympathy for women's and children's issues. (In fact, she tells me that as a child she used to collect stickers to give to her future pediatric patients.) As a member of XYZ Network at MIT, she was instrumental in promoting health education for our women.

Clara Barton is distinguished in many ways, and clearly she is a very outstanding candidate for medical school admission. Aside from her great academic talents, she has a tremendous curiosity and a flair with people. As a premedical advisor for the past 13 years as well as medical school faculty, I have had contact with many advisees and medical students. Ms. Barton is a member of the most outstanding six premedical advisees I have counseled, and I would enjoy being her attending in pediatrics. She should be offered admission to the most competitive schools.

Establishing a Relationship with Your Premedical Advisor

In all probability, your premedical advisor is a busy person with many things to do. If you want to foster a better relationship, try adhering to some of the following recommendations:

1. Arrive at your appointments on time. Bring copies of any material that your advisor should have. Do not expect your advisor to make the copies.
2. It is to your advantage to get to know your advisor. If your advisor is willing, find the time for an extra appointment or two.
3. Be very honest with your advisor. If you are having any special problems, or if there are issues concerning your application, tell your advisor. Any dishonesty will come back to haunt you, and may well destroy your chances for admission to medical school.
4. Feel free to ask your advisor questions. He or she probably has ready access to the answers or, at the minimum, knows how to find the answers.
5. Before submitting your personal statement to the medical schools, share it with your advisor. It is always helpful to have another person read the essays. I have had a number of students send me essays with serious grammatical errors as well as content issues. I do not believe that these essays would have been look at favorably by medical school admissions committees.
6. After hearing from medical schools, let your advisor know where you were accepted, where you were rejected, and what schools placed you on their waiting list. These will be listed in your record, and they may help your advisor with future students. It is also very thoughtful to write your advisor after you have attended medical school for a period of time and discuss the appropriateness of the school you selected and thank him/her for their help.

References — Chapter Three

---

1. Stewart, B.Y., "The Threatened Role of the Premedical Advisor," *Academic Medicine,* 68:547–548, 1993.
2. Lipman, Z.B., "Premedical Advising," *Journal of Medical Education,* 53:787–788, 1978.

Chapter Four

· · · · · · · · ·

THE APPLICATION PROCESS

For me, there was never really any doubt. By the time I was old enough to even think about careers, I knew that one day I would become a physician. In elementary school, I would daydream about the day I would wear a long white coat. Above the breast level pocket were the italicized words *Dr. Mark Goldstein, Department of Pediatrics.*

Thus, you should not be surprised that I began to read medical school admission material while I was still in high school. I wanted to be absolutely confident that I enrolled in all the required classes and completed all the necessary requirements.

Please do not feel that you must follow my example. It is certainly not necessary to start so early. On the other hand, procrastination or delay could seriously impair your chances for admission. When applying to medical school, timing remains a crucial element.

I instruct my premedical advisees to begin the application process in the middle of their junior year. That is the time, I tell them, they should register to take the MCAT and ask the appropriate people to write letters of reference. They should also read *Medical School Admission Requirements,* an annually revised guidebook published by the Association of American Medical Colleges (AAMC). The book has a good synopsis of each of the 125 medical schools in the U.S., and it includes information on Canadian medical schools. With the help of the book, students should develop long lists of prospective medical schools.

Competing pressures

· · · · · · · · · · · · · · ·

tempt one to believe that an

· · · · · · · · · · · · · · ·

issue deferred is a problem

· · · · · · · · · · · · · · ·

avoided; more often it is a

· · · · · · · · · · · · · · ·

crisis invented.

Henry Kissinger

A few months later, when the advisee and I have our end of the junior year meeting, we will have in our hands the MCAT scores, the final grades for the first three years of college, and the student's potential medical school list. Working together, the student and I will select at least 15 schools. My personal philosophy is to encourage candidates to apply to a small number of schools which are likely beyond his or her reach and some schools that are likely within reach. Most schools should be somewhere in-between. These determinations are often very difficult and require some frank discussions.

All students should apply to their state medical school. Since state schools frequently give preference to state residents, they are usually the schools that are most within reach for the typical candidate. On the other hand, schools which have been designated by the *U.S. News & World Report* to be among the top ten in the U.S. are beyond the reach of most applicants.

Once the list of medical schools has been compiled, the candidate should complete all necessary application forms. This is not as easy as it sounds. Only a small fraction of medical schools rely solely on the standard American Medical College Application Service (AMCAS) form. The vast majority of medical schools require applicants to complete a combination of forms. According to Richard I. Emmett, M.P.A., Associate Director of The Acadia Institute and the Medical College of Pennsylvania Medical Education Project and Assistant to the President, The Acadia Institute, Bar Harbor, Maine, with respect to application forms, medical schools may be divided into five different groups.

Fifteen medical schools — 12 percent — use only the AMCAS form. Seventeen medical schools — 14 percent — use only the school's own application form. Sixty-four schools, 51 percent, use both the AMCAS form and the school's own application form. Three schools use the AMCAS form or the AMCAS form plus supplemental forms for applicants to special programs. For example, the University of California–Los Angeles School of Medicine, requires applicants to its UCLA/Drew Joint Medical Program to complete the AMCAS and the school's own supplemental forms.

Meanwhile, Emmett notes, 27 schools — 21 percent — use the AMCAS form as one of two methods of preliminary screening. In the active screening method, schools use the information on the AMCAS form to make their initial cuts in the applicant pool. Only those applicants who are considered better candidates for admission will be sent the supplemental forms. In the passive screening method, which is believed to be less common, one of two letters is sent to those who have completed the AMCAS. The first letter informs the applicant that his or her credentials are not as competitive as most other applicants, thereby discouraging the submission of a supplemental application. Luckier candidates receive a second letter which indicates their application is still under consideration. They are told to complete the supplemental forms.

Emmett categorized the "extensiveness" of applications used by medical schools into three groups. The majority — 58 percent — use the AMCAS or forms that are analogous to the AMCAS. Twenty-five percent of the applications were "slightly to minimally more extensive than AMCAS." And, 17 percent were "moderately to significantly more extensive than AMCAS."

The extensiveness of applications was most apparent when the schools required essay responses to certain questions. Emmett contends that schools use these questions "to gauge a prospective student's possession of or potential to develop the personal qualities, values, attitudes, and attributes that both medical educators and the general public deem desirable in today's physician."

A content analysis completed on application essays from the schools that were "moderately to significantly more extensive than AMCAS" displayed two principal areas of interest. Almost half of the schools were oriented toward primary care. In their materials, they emphasized primary medicine, caring for underserved populations, and a concern for community health issues. And they asked applicants for information about the communities in which they spent their preundergraduate years. According to "Primary Care Task Force, Report of the Medical School Section," the communities where students lived during their preundergraduate years were an important factor associated with the choice of a career in primary care or the probability of practicing in an underserved area. The other area of interest was religion. Three of the schools with religious affiliations requested information that reflected a distinct religious orientation.

As part of the application process, medical schools requested other materials. While a current photograph was required by 54 schools, photographs were optional at 14 schools. No photograph was required by 58 schools. Forty-two schools requested information on criminal or felony convictions, and 22 schools wanted to know about any academic disciplinary action. Two schools required disclosure forms from undergraduate institutions. Six schools had a statement concerning the use of controlled drugs, and four schools had questions on mental health history or mental disabilities. Three schools asked for honor code statements. One school required applicants to report if they carried an infectious disease.

Each medical school has a designated committee on admissions. The committee may be headed by a physician or a nonphysician administrator. Typically, the committee consists of a number of physicians, preclinical faculty, and some medical students, as well as administrative personnel. Although other members of a school's faculty or staff may be involved in interviewing potential candidates for admission, not all of these are members of the admissions committee.

Letters of Recommendation

Letters of recommendation form a very important part of the application. Take extra time when considering those you will ask to write these letters. Be absolutely certain that you select people who will draft a positive piece that demonstrates insight and sensitivity.

It is my belief that applicants should have one or two letters from professors, a letter from a research advisor, and a letter from the premedical advisor. The premedical advisor letter is, by far, the most important. As noted in Chapter Three, some schools have a committee which writes the letter in the entirety; other schools have the premedical advisor write the letter for the council.

An added plus is to have a letter of reference written by an individual who is known to members of an admissions committee. This letter will likely have more influence than a letter written by an unknown reference.

Though it is sometimes assumed that letters from nonacademic individuals, members of the clergy, fraternity brothers, employment supervisors, and others play a strong role in the application process, I think they have little or no value. Do not waste your time on them.

Students have the right to inspect their letters of reference. However, *I am against this practice.* I suggest that students waive their rights to read their letters of reference by signing a copy of the Family Educational Rights and Privacy Act of 1994. While the knowledge that what I write will be reviewed by my advisees has not affected the content of my letters, other advisors have indicated that they are far more comfortable when students sign the waiver. Some faculty will write more superficial letters if they know the student will be reading them.

It should be noted that letters of recommendation must be written in a timely manner. Theoretically, most of the letter writing should take place in the spring or summer. However, many faculty members do not work in the summer. So it is very important to encourage, *diplomatically,* your references to write the letters in the spring — before the end of the school year. I emphasize *diplomati-*

cally for some important reasons. Obviously, you should not become an incessant nag. That could result in ill will. At the same time, your application to medical schools could be delayed if your file is incomplete. At MIT, all letters are mailed in one package. If one letter is missing, the entire package is held. Don't let a late letter of recommendation jeopardize your chances for admission.

While I request that each advisee supply me with an up-to-date resume or curriculum vitae, letters of recommendation should **not** be a simple summary of achievements. The most valuable letters are not a chronology of facts. Frequently, these facts have already been listed in the transcript, the AMCAS, or a supplementary application. Rather, the best letters describe the individual candidate and why he or she would be an asset to the medical school. Sometimes, I find it useful to rank the student — noting how the student compares to current and previous students.

Late Spring — Early Summer

After the meeting in June in which my advisee and I have formulated a semi-definite list of prospective medical schools, I tell my advisees to write the personal statement or essay for the AMCAS application. (This statement is so important that it will be discussed in far greater detail in Chapter Six, The Personal Statement.) During June and early July, I review these personal statements and help the students rework them. With my assistance, they are able to present themselves as valuable candidates who have much to contribute to the field of medicine. By mid-July, all of the essential elements of the AMCAS application should have been completed, and it should be mailed. With your classes over, you need to devote extra time to these undertakings. They are a crucial part of the process. Don't rush them.

While 88 medical schools participate in the Early Decision Program, it has never been popular with my advisees. Regardless, there are clear advantages to applying early. Since a candidate may apply early to only one medical school, it reduces the time required to complete applications, the time and money necessary to visit schools, and the unrelenting stress associated with the entire application process. However, it does require that a student decide at a very early date what medical school he or she would like to attend. And when the student is admitted, the offer must be accepted.

Some students believe that it is easier to obtain admission to a medical school through the early decision process. According to

Carol L. Elam, Ed.D., *et. al.*, an Assistant Dean for Admission at the University of Kentucky College of Medicine, this is a fallacy. Over a nine year period, Elam compared 839 early decision and regular admission matriculants to the University of Kentucky College of Medicine. As measured by the science and nonscience GPA, MCAT scores, and interview ratings, the early decision students had higher preadmission qualifications and were therefore a stronger pool of applicants compared to the regular admission applicants. During the first three years of medical school, the early decision students had higher GPAs.

Ideally, no later than July 15, the AMCAS application has been mailed and secondary application materials ("secondaries") are arriving from some medical schools. For non-AMCAS schools, application materials should have been requested. Since most students took the MCAT in the spring, they now have the time to complete the secondaries. The fall and winter should be reserved for interviews.

This is also the time to be attentive to details. All application documents, including primaries and secondaries, must be sent in a timely manner. If you change your address, notify AMCAS and those schools that do not participate in AMCAS. If you are invited for an interview, respond promptly. Notify all medical schools how you may be reached by either letter or telephone. And when you decide which medical school you will attend, withdraw you applications from the other schools. If you are lucky enough to receive two or more offers, accept the school you prefer and inform the other(s) of your decision.

References — Chapter Four

1. Emmett, R.I., "A Descriptive Analysis of Medical School Application Forms," *Academic Medicine,* 68:564–569, 1993.
2. "Primary Care Task Force, Report of the Medical School Section," *JAMA,* 268:1092, 1992.
3. Elam, C.L., Johnson, M.M.S., "Front Door or Back Door: Comparison of Preadmission and Medical School Performances of Early-decision and Regular-admission Students," *Academic Medicine,* S:60–62, 1994.

Chapter Five

THE MEDICAL COLLEGE ADMISSION TEST (MCAT)

In 1967, when I took the Medical College Admission Test (MCAT), I did not enroll in any review courses or pour over stacks of review books. Why? The answer is simple. There were no such offerings.

But that was not my only problem. Unlike today's students, who receive their MCAT score a few months after the tests are administered, when I was in school, we never learned the test results. We had absolutely no way of determining how we fared. Could we enjoy a momentary minisigh of relief knowing we had obtained a top score or was it time to begin worrying that our results were far from spectacular? Even worse, had we done so poorly that a full-fledged panic was in order? Thank goodness, things are so different now. If students so desire, they may participate in review courses and read a host of review books. And, while the wait may seem long to the students, in reality, the MCAT results are processed very quickly.

The MCAT has been ***the*** medical school admission test for decades. According to the Association of American Medical Colleges (AAMC), the MCAT is a standardized, multiple-choice examination used by admissions committees to predict the future performance of medical school applicants. It provides admissions committees with standardized measures of academic performance for all examinees under equivalent conditions. The test is developed by a number of different individuals including medical school admissions officers, premedical instructors, medical educators, physicians, the AAMC, and other experts.

It takes 20 years to make an overnight success.

Eddie Cantor

The AAMC maintains that by testing students in scientific and nonscientific disciplines the MCAT encourages students interested in a medical career to pursue a broad undergraduate education, not only in science and social science but also in humanities. The MCAT assesses scientific problem-solving, critical thinking, written communication, and the ability to understand concepts of medical science.

The AAMC administers the MCAT on a Saturday, twice yearly, in April and August. Previously, it had been offered in April and September. But when applicants took the tests in September, their scores were not released until November. And since some medical schools do not make admission decisions without results from the MCAT, those students had a decided disadvantage.

Applicants are expected to take the MCAT 18 months prior to medical school matriculation. For applicants who are unable to take the test on a Saturday — due to unavoidable conflicts or religious beliefs — there is provision for special Sunday testing. The AAMC must be notified in advance. Most medical schools and premedical advisors prefer applicants to take the exam in April. This allows for a timely release of scores. Generally, there is very little course content that will be presented between April and August that would help the applicant achieve a higher score.

The MCAT has four sections — verbal reasoning, physical sciences, biological sciences, and the writing sample. Verbal reasoning is designed to measure the ability of the applicant to understand, evaluate, and apply information and arguments to prose text. It draws upon material an applicant would have learned in humanities, social science, and natural science courses. Specific subject matter is not tested. All the necessary facts are presented in the passage the applicant evaluates.

The physical sciences section appraises the ability of the applicant to understand basic concepts and solve problems in the area of physics and physically-related chemistry. It covers specifics that should have been taught in undergraduate courses in inorganic and organic chemistry and noncalculus physics. This section consists entirely of science problems, including elements presented in graphs, tables, and charts.

The biological sciences subtest assesses the understanding of basic biological concepts and facility in solving problems in the area of biology and biologically related chemistry. The background for this section comes from general biology courses. This part also has problems and data presented in graphs, tables, and charts.

The final section, the writing sample, is a measure of the applicant's ability to develop and synthesize concepts of a central idea, and it is an evaluation of the capability of presenting this idea in a clear, logical, and cohesive manner. It is expected that the grammar, syntax, and punctuation will be consistent with the first draft of a composition.

The writing sample is administered at the beginning of the afternoon testing session. Applicants have 60 minutes to compose two essays — 30 minutes on each theme. The essay topics do not pertain to the technical content of biology, chemistry, physics, or mathematics. Nor do they relate to the medical school application process or the specific reasons for choosing medicine as a potential career. Obscure social or cultural issues and religious or emotionally charged concerns are not presented.

According to the Princeton Review book *Cracking the MCAT 1995,* the following are examples of two essay questions:

A government cannot enforce a law if its citizens oppose it.

No false statement can live indefinitely.

As previously mentioned, there are now many books that may help students prepare for the MCAT. The AAMC publishes the *MCAT Student Manual* and the *Full Length MCAT Practice Test 1.* The *MCAT Student Manual* outlines the sections of the test and the content reasoning skills that they will evaluate. It also offers suggestions on how to prepare for the test. The *Full Length MCAT Practice Test 1* includes a released operational test from April 1991. The items in this booklet are similar to test materials used in an actual MCAT.

The scores on the verbal reasoning and physical and biological sciences tests range from one, the lowest, to 15, the highest. The expectation is that two medical school candidates of equal ability will achieve the same scaled score. Since the same scale is used for all three areas of assessment, comparisons may be made between the three sections. Such commonly scaled scores enable medical school admissions committees to compare students who have taken the tests at different times.

Scores on the writing sample are reported alphabetically from "J", the lowest, to "T", the highest. At least two different people read and score each writing sample. The score received represents their combined scores.

The AAMC reviewed 63,683 tests administered in April and August of 1994. For these 1994 test takers the mean scaled scores were as follows:

Verbal reasoning   7.8
Physical sciences   8.0
Biological sciences   8.0
Writing sample   The 50th percentile was "N"

In the verbal reasoning, as well as the physical, and biological sciences portions of the test, the ninetieth-and-above percentile was achieved at the scaled score of 11. With the writing sample, the ninetieth-and-above percentile score was at the test level of "R".

What is a good MCAT score? There is no clear answer. It is generally believed that a score of ten or higher on the subtests and "Q" on the writing sample are quite reasonable. However, these scores must be weighed against many other factors in the applicant's file such as the applicant's overall preparation for medical school, grades in courses, and the competitiveness of the college attended.

Should you retake the test if your scores are not at the level you would have liked? Although this is a question that should be discussed with your premedical advisor, there are several important reasons why the test should be retaken. However, if there is an unusual difference between your scores and college grades, if you took the test before completing your introductory courses, if you had a serious illness on the day of the test, or if your premedical advisor suggests you repeat the test, it would probably be to your advantage to take the MCAT again.

Will participation in a MCAT preparatory course significantly improve your scores? If the only intervening variable between your first test and your retest is such further coursework in the field, more than likely your retest will not show a markedly better score.

You might be interested in an AAMC study of examinees who tested in April 1993, and once prior to that. Of the examinees who received a ten in the verbal reasoning portion of the first test, only 32 percent improved with the retest. If the score was 11, only nine percent increased their score in subsequent testing.

Of those who received a score of nine on the biological science subtest, 43 percent gained one or more points on the retest, 30 percent had no change, and 28 percent had a lower score. Of those who earned a score of 12, 16 percent scored one or two points higher on the retest, 56 percent lost one or more points, and 28 percent did not change. It is apparent that for the biological sciences subtest, the likelihood of increasing your score diminishes significantly if your initial score is 11 or more.

When students had lower scores on the first biological science test, the situation was quite different. If a student received a score of five on the first test, then on retest 66 percent of the students increased their scores. Interestingly, on the physical sciences test, only 31 percent of those scoring ten on the first test improved with retesting. And, with the writing sample section, 42 percent of those who had received an "O" on their first sample, earned a higher score when retested.

There is another way to evaluate the data. Examinees who scored a ten in their first verbal reasoning subtest had an average retested score change of –.27. Those who received a ten in their first biological sciences subtest experienced a – .02 change with retesting. For physical sciences examinees who initially earned a ten, the average score change was –.18. Examinees who achieved scores of "N", "O", or "P" in the writing sample, had a zero average change when retested. These data suggest that examinees who earn scores of ten in the subtests should not, in most cases, repeat the test. And unless there is a significant reason, those who earn "N", "O", "P", "Q", "S", or "T" on the writing sample should also not repeat the test.

On the other hand, if initial test scores on the verbal reasoning, physical, or biological sciences were one through nine, then an average positive score change was achieved by applicants taking the MCAT for a second time. And if the first result of the writing sample was "J", "K", "L", or "M", then about half of all applicants improved one or more letters.

According to *Facts,* a publication prepared by the Section for Student Services of the AAMC, the following are the mean MCAT scores for all of the 46,591 students applying to medical school in 1995:

Verbal reasoning	8.5
Physical sciences	8.6
Writing sample	"O"
Biological sciences	8.7

The mean scores for all of the 16,253 matriculants in 1995 were as follows:

Verbal reasoning	9.5
Physical sciences	9.7
Writing sample	"P"
Biological sciences	9.8

At the 1994 AAMC Annual Meeting, George A. Nowacek, Ph.D., Director of Educational Research and Development at the Medical

College of Ohio in Toledo, discussed his research on the relationship between MCAT scores and medical school achievement. For his study, Nowacek chose 16 different medical schools and followed classes entering in 1992 and 1993. Nowacek found that the first year of medical school Grade Point Average (GPA) was more strongly correlated with the MCAT than with the undergraduate GPA.

Another study was completed on the first year GPA of classes entering 13 medical schools in 1992. Not surprisingly, it found that students with the highest undergraduate GPAs and MCAT scores who attend the more selective colleges earn higher GPAs during their first year of medical school. And an investigation of students in four medical schools found that there was a much stronger relationship between the score on the biological sciences portion of the MCAT and the grade earned in medical school microbiology than the score on the writing sample and the grade in the same microbiology class. In fact, the scores on the writing sample section had very little correlation with achievement in any first year medical school courses. It appears that when predicting first year medical school GPA, the most important MCAT subtest is biological sciences.

It is worth noting that Nowacek also found very little improvement when the MCAT was repeated. According to Nowacek, the average point increase in most MCAT retests was approximately one half of a point. Nowacek commented that it was possible that this increase is related to coaching or practice.

Robert F. Jones, Ph.D., a Research Associate in the Division of Educational Measurement and Research of the AAMC, and Maria Thomae-Forgues, a Human Resource Specialist at the Organization of American States, found that the "MCAT scores by themselves have significant predictive validity with respect to first and second year medical school course grades and National Board of Medical Examiners Part I examination scores and that they complement the predictive validity of undergraduate college grades."

Table 5-1 shows the average 1992 MCAT scores for applicants **accepted** to medical school.

Table 5-2 reviews the MCAT performance by racial/ethnic group for the April 1995 test.

While several minorities score lower on the MCAT test, it should be noted that they are accepted with their lower scores. This will be discussed further in Chapter Eight — Minority Students.

One final thought. Some basic science undergraduate courses at some undergraduate schools do not adequately prepare students for the MCAT subtests. While some schools design their basic sci-

	Verbal Reasoning	Physical Sciences	Biological Sciences	Writing Sample (median score)

Table 5-1
MCAT Scores for Applicants Accepted to Medical School

	Verbal Reasoning	Physical Sciences	Biological Sciences	Writing Sample (median score)
Black	7.4	6.9	7.2	O
American Indian	8.5	7.4	8.0	O
Mexican American	8.3	7.8	8.3	O
Mainland Puerto Rican	7.9	7.6	7.9	O
White	9.6	9.4	9.5	O
Asian	9.2	10.1	9.9	O
Commonweath Puerto Rican	5.7	6.7	7.1	N
Other Hispanic	9.1	8.7	8.9	O

Source: Minority Student Opportunities In United States Medical Schools 1993–1994 *published by Association of American Medical Colleges.*

ence courses to ensure higher results in the MCAT subtests, others do not. Check with your premedical advisory office to determine your school's overall average for the MCAT subtests. You may find that the mean score in certain subtests is at or below the national average for all test takers.

If your basic science courses have not sufficiently prepared you for the MCAT, make the time for additional study. There are several books on the market which may be of assistance. Additionally, it is useful to know that admissions committees are aware that students from some schools do not score as well in certain MCAT subtests. Furthermore, some admissions committees concurrently review the application materials of all candidates from the same school. Thus, the MCAT scores are evaluated in the context of the same undergraduate preparation.

The Table 5-3 indicates the April 1995 MCAT performance by the undergraduate major of the individual taking the test. Finally, the age of the individual taking the test with breakdown of subtest scores is presented in Table 5-4. This table demonstrates that as the student ages, MCAT subtest scores decline modestly.

In summation, the MCAT, which is a requirement for all applicants to medical school, is considered to be an objective criterion used to measure all applicants against one another. Preferably, it

Table 5-2
April 1995 MCAT Performance by Racial/Ethnic Group

Race/Ethnic Group	Number	Verbal Reasoning	Physical Sciences	Biological Sciences	Writing Sample
White	18,287	8.4 (2.2)	8.3 (2.2)	8.6 (2.2)	O
Black	2,085	5.8 (2.3)	5.8 (1.9)	5.9 (2.3)	N
Mexican American/ Chicano	578	7.0 (2.4)	7.0 (2.1)	7.4 (2.2)	O
American Indian/ Alaskan Native	200	7.5 (2.3)	7.1 (2.2)	7.2 (2.2)	N
Mainland Puerto Rican	189	6.1 (2.8)	6.4 (2.4)	6.5 (2.7)	M
Commonwealth Puerto Rican	407	3.9 (1.9)	5.0 (1.6)	4.9 (2.2)	J
Asian/Pacific Islander	5,992	7.5 (2.4)	8.5 (2.4)	8.7 (2.3)	O
Other Hispanic	632	7.4 (2.4)	7.5 (2.2)	7.8 (2.4)	O
Underrepresented Minority	3,052	6.2 (2.4)	6.3 (2.4)	6.1 (2.1)	N
Other Minority	7,031	7.3 (2.6)	8.4 (2.5)	8.2 (2.5)	O

Source: Association of American Medical Colleges.
Number scores represent mean values with standard deviation in parentheses. Letter scores represent median values.

should be taken in April of the year prior to entrance to medical school when applicants should have completed all of their required coursework. The scores are an important — but not the most important — criterion for admission to medical school. Scores of ten or higher on the subtests and "O" on the writing sample generally indicate that the test should not be repeated. Test repeaters often do not have notable gains in their scores. While coaching or preparatory courses are common, it is unclear whether they result in score increases. Certainly, self-study using materials prepared by various organizations or the AAMC may be of assistance and will familiarize students with the types of questions they will be asked.

Table 5-3
April 1995 MCAT Performance by Undergraduate Major

Undergraduate Major	Number	Verbal Reasoning	Physical Sciences	Biological Sciences	Writing Sample
Math & Statistics	231	8.1 (2.7)	8.9 (2.6)	8.4 (2.7)	O
Specialized Health Services	1,613	6.9 (2.5)	6.9 (2.2)	7.2 (2.4)	N
Biological Sciences	17,219	7.7 (2.4)	8.0 (2.3)	8.4 (2.4)	O
Humanities	1,125	9.0 (2.3)	8.4 (2.2)	8.5 (2.3)	P
Physical Sciences	4,103	8.0 (2.5)	9.2 (2.5)	8.6 (2.4)	O
Social Sciences	3,361	8.4 (2.3)	7.9 (2.2)	8.1 (2.3)	P
Other	2,273	8.2 (2.6)	8.1 (2.5)	8.2 (2.6)	O

Source: Association of American Medical Colleges (AAMC).
Number scores represent mean values with standard deviation in parentheses. Letter scores represent median values.

Table 5-4
April 1995 MCAT Performance by Applicant's Age

Age	Number	Verbal Reasoning	Physcial Sciences	Biological Sciences	Writing Sample
<21	1,322	8.4 (2.4)	9.0 (2.5)	9.0 (2.4)	O
21–22	15,520	8.1 (2.3)	8.3 (2.3)	8.5 (2.3)	O
23–27	9,362	7.6 (2.5)	7.8 (2.3)	8.1 (2.4)	O
28–31	2,007	7.6 (2.6)	7.8 (2.5)	7.9 (2.5)	N
>31	1,714	7.4 (2.8)	7.4 (2.5)	7.5 (2.6)	N

Source: Association of American Medical Colleges (AAMC).
Number scores represent mean values with standard deviation in parentheses. Letter scores represent median values.

References — Chapter Five

1. *Medical School Admission Requirements 1996–97,* Association of American Medical Colleges, 1995.
2. *Cracking The MCAT 1995 Edition,* The Princeton Review, 1994.
3. "Explanation of Scores for Advisors," Association of American Medical Colleges," MCAT, 1994.
4. MCAT Summary Data, NAAHP Annual Meeting, June, 1994.
5. *Facts,* Association of American Medical Colleges, 1994.
6. Nowacek, G.A., "MCAT Predictive Validity Research Study," Presented at the Annual Meeting, Association of American Medical Colleges, 1994.
7. Jones, R.F., Thomae-Forgues, M., "Validity of the MCAT in Predicting Performance In the First Two Years of Medical School," *Journal of Medical Education,* 59:455–464, 1984.
8. *Minority Student Opportunities In United States Medical Schools, 1993–94, 12th Edition,* Association of American Medical Colleges, 1993.
9. Personal Communication, Association of American Medical Colleges, 1995.

Chapter Six
. . . .

THE PERSONAL STATEMENT

The AMCAS application requires all candidates to write a personal statement. This statement or essay enables students to explain why they have selected medicine as a career. It also provides a forum to discuss some extracurricular or work-related accomplishments.

But the statement has the potential to do much more. For example, it may be used by a candidate to explain perceived weaknesses in an application. Thus, if there is a notable reason (such as an illness or death in the family) why an applicant did poorly in a course, it may be addressed in the statement.

> *The difference between the right word and the almost right word is the difference between lightning and the lighting bug.*
>
> **Mark Twain**

Over the years, in my capacity as a pre-medical advisor, I have reviewed scores of statements. From my experience, I would like to offer the following suggestions.

◆ Before you begin writing, determine the message or messages you wish to convey. Outlining your thoughts is often helpful.

◆ Begin the statement with a catchy line — something that will grab and hold the reader's attention. By the end of the first few sentences, the reader should be very anxious to read more.

◆ Make the statement interesting. A dull statement will not be read closely. At best, it may be skimmed. More likely, after the first boring paragraph it will be put aside.

◆ Do not use the statement to reiterate achievements noted elsewhere in your application. There is nothing more monotonous than reading a litany of facts that have already been listed.

- Write your statement in much the same way that you would write a letter to a friend. The best statements read as if a conversation is taking place between the writer and the reader. Avoid a formal or stilted style. When appropriate, humor, anecdotal material, and rich details are welcome additions. Some students use a painful experience, such as a serious illness or death in the family, to explain why they are interested in medicine.
- Project your personal qualities that may not be ascertained from other parts of the written application. For example, qualities such as leadership, altruism, scientific curiosity, and compassion may be developed and expanded through the use of illustrations.
- Be certain your essay shows you as a unique person. You must stand out from the crowd of applicants. After reviewing the essay, the reader should have a memorable picture of you.
- While you should write your own statement, have it reviewed by others. Particular attention should be paid to grammar, syntax, and spelling. Almost every draft I have read has had serious problems with construction. If these statements had been submitted, they may very well have impaired the chances for admission. Members of the admissions committee could have questioned the written communication skills of these applicants.
- Review your statement many times. Don't wait until the last minute. Rewrite and then rewrite again.

One other hint. Some students use different fonts which allow more words per page. Using a smaller font allows more words per page than a bigger font. However, I suggest you use a standard size font so that your statement is easily read. The AMCAS application requires that the entire statement fit on one page.

The following samples of personal statements are from my MIT advisees who have been admitted to one or more U.S. medical schools. I have attempted to present a variety of statements demonstrating some of the previously outlined techniques. The statements vary in length and the central elements of each statement are highlighted.

Statement #1

- A catchy first sentence
- A good explanation of why this student switched to premed late in her college career

John Smith, a young man from Norway afflicted with Cystic Fibrosis, wanted to run the New York City Marathon. As an extension of my involvement with a track club for disabled persons, I ran with him as a volunteer escort and supporter. During the marathon I encouraged him, pointed out landmarks and attractions along the way, and engaged in light conversation. I was in high school at the time and I told him about my aspirations of becoming an oceanographer.

Having been born and raised in New York City, oceanography seemed mysterious to me and became a point of departure for my study of science. During the high school year, I became involved with the recovery program for the endangered Hawaiian Monk Seal. I had the opportunity to go to Honolulu where I cared for adult male seals before their transfer to aquariums and seaparks and I rehabilitated injured seal pups before their release into the ocean. I continued my involvement through college when I spent a summer in their natural habitat, Kure Atoll, a remote island in the Hawaiian chain. As one of two field workers, I was responsible for tagging seals and maintaining seal pups in pens. Another summer I was a research fellow at the Scripps Institution of Oceanography where I did work in geochemistry analyzing sediment to deduce ancient climate patterns. The following year, as a continuation of that work, I participated in a two week drilling cruise off of Mendocino, California. At MIT, I researched the chemical evolution of hydrothermal vents at the location of sea floor spreading. This past spring I dove, as the only undergraduate ever, in the submarine ALVIN, 2,800 meters below the ocean surface off of the Pacific Coast of Mexico. We sampled water from the hot springs for my analysis and collected the giant clams and tubeworms that proliferate around the vents.

I feel fortunate to have studied oceanography as my beginning in science. My experience with John Smith reminds me, though, that my most significant and rewarding experiences have always involved helping people. It is my interaction with people that gives me sustained fulfillment and satisfaction. Throughout college I have been drawn to similar pursuits in which I can advise and help people including my roles as captain of the women's and coach of the freshman sailing teams, associate freshman advisor and teaching assistant, big sister of my living group, and leader of a forum for freshman on health issues at MIT.

I find my current work at the Adolescent Medicine Clinic of the Boston Children's Hospital, where I serve as peer counselor and observer especially interesting and rewarding. At the clinic I meet with underprivileged urban youths and I counsel them on safe sexual practices. Many of the teens are similar to my schoolmates from the New York City public school system and I find I can relate to their concerns. I appreciate the interaction I have with them, as well as their humor and their candor. In addition to the patients, I interact with the attending physician, fellow, resident, and medical students and I enjoy being part of a medical team. This experience has been invaluable because it has exposed me to a career that involves all of my interests. To me, medicine represents the elegant balance of human interaction, social duty, and intellectual stimulation.

Medicine appeals to me because of the direct and immediate impact it can have on people's lives. The clinic is a submarine into inner-city society. Yet at the clinic I can be more than an observer; I have the opportunity not only to study, but to effect change. Adolescent medicine captivates me because it allows me to effect this change at a very critical period of development. I feel purposeful and eager to serve at the clinic. And while the result may be unpredictable, the work is deeply satisfying. Although I often come home physically and emotionally haggard, I am always certain that there is nothing else I'd rather be doing.

Statement # 2

- ◆ Excellent first sentence
- ◆ Description of a long-standing interest in medicine
- ◆ Explanation of interest in pediatrics

When I was five years old, I touched a cow's eye. This initial interest in medicine occurred during a demonstration of optical anatomy at a museum in San Francisco. I was the lone volunteer to step forward and touch the eye. A stranger standing in the back row observed to my parents, "She's a natural." My desire to become a physician was strengthened during Anatomy and Physiology class in high school. The dissection of the brain and spinal cord of my cat in one piece — no one had accomplished this task before — reinforced my ambition.

My strong commitment to assisting others stems from my previous experiences working with children. My first experience was in junior high school as a volunteer swimming instructor at the town park. In high school, I volunteered for four years as an assistant dance teacher to children in my community. Not only did I spend many hours a week teaching aspiring ballerinas how to arabesque, I was instrumental in organizing an annual dance marathon which raised money for the American Heart Association. As I entered college, I enhanced these experiences by volunteering at Children's Hospital in Boston. My assignment consisted of feeding, playing, or simply reading to terminally ill children. I was touched by many of the children, but I especially remember an orphan, Sara, whose sole desire was to play dolls with someone. When I returned to visit her one week and was informed that she had succumbed to her illness, I was shocked by my strong feelings of grief. Her image remains with me even today.

As these various experiences strengthened my desire to work with children, I sought and obtained a research position in Pediatrics and Public Health. This experience differed from my previous technical research positions in the fields of chemistry and biology, and helped me realize my goal to be a clinician rather than a researcher. From my experience in the Joint Program for Neonatology (JPN) at Children's Hospital, I have discovered that the skills required of a physician are broad and complex: clinical, ethical, analytical, and technical. Participating in the JPN has allowed me to take a valuable look at the analysis of medical data and the techniques that go into patient care. Additionally, my current study of maternal health and persistent pulmonary hypertension of the newborn and my previous work with bronchopulmonary dysplasia have enabled me to observe various aspects of medicine not available in technical laboratories such as the importance of communication and medical ethics when dealing with patients. In addition to my work in public health, my involvement in the JPN summer intern program for the past two summers has allowed me to observe cesarean sections as part of the triage team, and participate in mock diagnosis and treatment of patients. I have also had the unique opportunity to perform the Brazelton exam for Newborns with R. Berry Brazelton.

A physician's life demands a balance between medical, family, and community responsibilities. At MIT, I have not only managed to balance stringent academic demands with various extracurricular activities, but I have planned my curriculum to be complete in three and one-half years so that I may continue my research in pediatrics and public health full-time in the spring of 1995. In addition, I have extended myself to the local community by volunteering for two years at Children's Hospital. All of these experiences have broadened my understanding of the doctor's role as society's healer and reinforced my dedication to become a physician.

Statement # 3

- ◆ Great first sentence
- ◆ Essay is interesting, personal, and convincing
- ◆ Writer sensitive to discomfort of patient
- ◆ Superb concluding paragraph

I think I was about eight when I first realized I had a secret. I was, and am, ignorant of the secret's origin and final outcome. Nevertheless, even as a proud eight-year-old owner I could tell even then that it was something spectacular. My secret is not something tangible. You can neither hold it in your hands nor examine it with your eyes. However, you can, or at least I can, feel it with the heart. It is a slue of mixed feelings intertwined with each other that together hold something wonderful. To grab hold and take advantage of my secret's wonders all that is needed is the key to unlock its splendor. Therein lied the problem. As an eight-year-old child, I neither possessed the key nor knew where to find it. A curious child as to the secret's contents, I tucked the secret away in a corner of my heart for safekeeping and began the search.

The first big hint as to the key's location came about two years later. It had been a particularly rough season for me and my asthma. I had frequented the hospital too much, and in this instance, too long. I was having difficulties breathing, nothing new, but this visit was different. The doctors were trying new medication and the side effects had increased in number and intensity. I remember lying perfectly still staring at my mother's face asking God to please take away some of the hurt when I inhaled a little too deeply inducing a coughing attack. When I was able to control the coughing, I turned to my mother and said, "Mom, I want to die."

I was a child who could not imagine it ever hurting that much; a child tired of fighting something she could not see nor understand; a child to whom death was only a means to stop the hurt. I was also a child who saw her mother cry in front of her for the first time. As I watched tears flow from her eyes I was overcome with feelings that by all logic should have been new and unexplored; yet, they were both warm and familiar. Confused, I looked deep into my mother's eyes searching for an explanation. What I saw was a glimpse of my secret.

In that brief moment I learned a great deal about life, and somehow that connected to my secret. I learned to understand death and the complex mixture of sorrow and release it brings. I realized how the people around me were trying each in their own way to help me. Even more importantly, I learned what their efforts, successful or not, meant. The efforts made by the doctors, nurses, and my family formed a connection between the world around me and myself. This connection seemed to tug on my heart as if to imply that this is where it belonged. I squeezed my mother's hand and looked into her eyes to let her know I understood. In so doing, I experienced the satisfying warm feeling that I am sure those helping me enjoyed. The feeling was incredible, addictive and again familiar. There was no doubt this was part of my secret.

With each passing year I glimpsed at my secret more frequently. Each time learning, or more appropriately, becoming conscious of something that it seemed some part of me already knew. For example, volunteering at a senior citizen's home I had a chance to share a dance with an elderly gentleman whose smile reminded me that a person's mere presence can work miracles. I had not realized until that moment how important it is to me to make a difference in the lives of people around me. I do not pretend to be a miracle worker, but somebody has got to care enough to try. My elderly friend not only taught me how to dance, but also started me on the path I am today. I was trying to answer his question as to why I choose to become an engineer when he suggested I try working with kids. It was his opinion that I would make a wonderful teacher. His advice and my love for children led me to volunteer at the Children's Hospital the past two summers.

I had completed my first year in college and declared a chemical engineering major. I enjoyed the material and was thus confident in my choice. I was not, however, prepared for what I would experience working with those kids. My time at the Children's Hospital was filled with so much. For example, when I could get a child to smile or laugh it felt as if the joy the child was experiencing translated directly into my reward. In essence, I was happy both with myself and what I was doing. It is simplistic, but it just felt right for me to be there. However, not as a volunteer that worked with the kids a couple of hours a day, but as a doctor who would be able to do so much more for them. It shocked me the first time I came to this realization at how comfortable it felt. There was no hesitation, simply affirmation that yes, this is who you are. I had found my secret's key or rather, the key had found me. As it turns out, the key was in my heart all along. My mistake was looking with my eyes when I should have been looking with my heart. I still do not pretend to completely understand my secret. I fathom that it will be a long time and many experiences later before I do. Medical school takes me one stop closer to that understanding. Being a doctor will take me one step closer to unraveling my secret's secret.

Statement # 4
- First paragraph outlines student's interest in medicine
- Very good explanation of why student wants to pursue a career in research instead of clinical medicine

My choice of medicine as a career was initially influenced by the circumstances that my family and I underwent since immigrating to the U.S. from China in 1979. In China, going to the doctor was not a problem. However, during the first few years in the U.S., the language obstacle and the consequent inconvenience of asking somebody to interpret prevented us from seeking medical help unless it was absolutely necessary. Since my father was not allowed to emigrate with the family until five years later, the fear of medical cost also deterred us. To lessen the burden of my family in situations of medical distress initially motivated me to become a doctor. I realized that other Chinese immigrant families must endure similar experiences. Hoping that my help would provide some comfort, I interpreted for relatives and family friends when they visited their doctors. Their words of gratitude aroused my compassion. More and more I felt compelled to become a doctor so that I can help in a more direct and effective way.

Knowing that the success of medicine results from not only humanistic but also scientific efforts, I further confirmed my interest in medicine by exploring medical research. During the summer of 1990, I volunteered in a biomolecular research laboratory under the supervision of Dr. XXX at Massachusetts General Hospital. I not only acquired various biomolecular techniques but also was first introduced to the atmosphere and demands of research work. Furthermore, working with Dr. XXX gave me the chance to learn about the schedule and nature of a doctor's work.

The satisfaction and knowledge that I gained from my summer job led me to pursue further research work at MIT. Therefore, in the spring of 1991, I assisted YYY, a Ph.D. candidate in chemical engineering, in the on-going study of biodegradable polymeric delivery devices used for vaccination. My responsibilities included making controlled release devices for BSA in mice to determine the effect of the adjuvant-active L-tyrosine-based polymer on the antibody response to releasing antigen, and tracking the immune response via the enzyme linked immunosorbent assay. This past summer, I began working in Prof. ZZZ's organic chemistry research group. I was responsible for resynthesizing the alphahelix template, an organic molecule that induces a helical formation in short peptides when attached by their N-termini. By understanding how proteins fold into their characteristic conformations, one can further study their functions as enzymes in the human body. From my research experiences, I realize how encompassing the field of medicine can be.

To me, the enrichments of a physician's work will come from participating in advancing research and the opportunity to use my skills and knowledge wherever I go and at any time. Moreover, I hope to provide a sense of security and dependability to all those around me. Medicine as a profession can transcend place, time, and race. Although I have been warned that medical studies are physically and mentally arduous, I feel that my education at MIT has taught and imbued me with perseverance, the key to reaching one's goal. The foremost satisfaction that I, as a doctor, will seek is the rewarding feeling in knowing that I have helped lessen the suffering of another human being.

Statement # 5

◆ A shocking opening statement
◆ Very well written essay that ties together in the last paragraph
◆ This statement illustrates how a student used a tragic situation to bring meaning to his own life

In the winter of 1990, the night before my Circuits and Electronics final, I received a phone call telling me that my high school friend, Darryl, had committed suicide. I was shocked, so overwhelmed by the news that I couldn't cry. Feeling both angry and deserted, I tried to imagine what could have gone so wrong that he would throw away what I thought was a good life. My fraternity brothers tried to understand what I felt, but even I couldn't understand what I was feeling. Still feeling numbness, I didn't perform very well on my final the next day, and I went home in a state of bewilderment.

Losing such a close friend made me realize how fragile life is, how meaningless it can be, and forced me to think about what I really wanted out of life. How important is being an engineer?

Could I leave any lasting impressions in this world? Up to this point in life, I was satisfied with attending my classes, working hard, and trying to get good grades; however, this episode made me face a startling reality; maybe life wasn't as simple as I thought it to be. Being an electrical engineer had been my life's dream since I played with electronic gadgets as a kid. But during the term following Darryl's death, the critical thinking that I did about my life caused me to wonder if I wasn't applying my abilities in a misdirected manner. For sure, I enjoyed engineering, but could there be something else, something higher than I was striving for?

I spent the summer following my sophomore year at Rockwell International, working on the instrumentation used to test both production and development hardware for the Space Shuttle main engine. The project that was to take me all summer only took two weeks to complete. My supervisors and all the engineers were very pleased with my progress, but the more I saw of the daily routines of an engineer, the more I knew that I did not want to be one for the rest of my life. All the circuit analysis, digital design, semiconductor theory, and signal analysis that I had been studying at MIT had been broken down into a series of writing reports and performing the same tests. Many of the engineers even told me that they did not use much of what they had learned in college. If that was the case, I couldn't do this for a career.

When I thought about why engineering had captured my interest, I told myself it was the problem solving aspect of it; observing a system, diagnosing the source of the problem, and knowing enough about the system in order to know how to correct it.

Although I believe that an undergraduate major in engineering is the best way to get an education in this critical thinking method, I know that a number of careers require this critical thinking and would make me happy, including medicine.

I have always had a keen interest in biology and medicine but had pushed it aside when I decided to become an engineer. Coming back to school for my junior year, I decided to pursue that interest, by finding a research position at the Boston Heart Foundation in Cambridge. During that term I created the computer lab at the facility; installing the computers and software, setting up the network, and dealing with hardware problems as they arose. Once that was completed, I assisted in teaching the doctors to use the system to collect data from angiograms. Next term my project will involve computer modelling of coronary blood vessels, and it will expand into my undergraduate thesis. This research position allows me to mix my engineering experience and interest in biology and medicine and has shown me that while engineering and medicine may be two dissimilar fields, they complement each other well.

As the goal of becoming a doctor materialized in my head, this new sense of purpose drove me to excel both in school and my most important extracurricular activity, my fraternity. After all the experiences that I've share with my brothers, I feel obligated to them. Whether it is pulling an all-nighter to work on the Rush Book and then going to install a chapter at Harvard the next morning or just caring enough to help out a brother in a class, each act of sharing that I give helps bring our house closer together. Certainly it is difficult to look after others when so many of my own problems fill my head, but anyone can be helpful and think about others when he has the time. The true test of brotherhood is the service that I give to others when I find myself needing it the most. To know that I can make my brothers feel a closer brotherhood because of me, means that I have a duty to work hard to make it so. And when they put enough trust in my abilities to elect me to be President and Rush Chairman, two very important offices, in the same term, I know that I will work just as hard in the future.

Although mixing a busy extracurricular schedule and academics made for many sleepless nights, the desire that I had to pursue medicine seriously drove me to tackle even more. The next term I kept on with my interests, and was happily rewarded to see that I did well in my biology course and bioelectronics laboratory class. They came easier to me than my previous courses because I loved what I was doing and my interest in the subject had a more defined purpose.

This summer, I'm taking a developmental biology course at UCLA and volunteering at the UCI Medical Center, in addition to working at Gish Biomedical Inc. and running our fraternity's Rush program. I am truly excited to experience the clinical application of medicine, and the biology class is to be certain that I enjoy the academic nature of the field that will consume me for at least the next four years. Working in the payroll department at Gish doesn't expose me to much of the actual biomedical work, but I often sneak down to the production floor to watch the manufacturing of the equipment that I see so often at the hospital and at my research project.

Working at the Medical Center is the happiest thing I could possibly be doing. Assisting doctors in the ER to place a cast on a teenager, or to help drain fluid from a man's knee, this is the first experience that I've had to clinical medicine, and I am drawn to it. I've seen a gunshot victim close to death, and I've also had the joy of seeing a patient's family smile and hug him as I wheel him out of the recovery room. And when that patient got out of his wheelchair, shook my hand, and said thanks before getting into his car, I knew that was the reason I wanted to get into medicine. It's been a long time since that winter vacation, when my high school friends and I went to visit Darryl's grave. I think about how different our lives are now; two years of college sure have changed a lot about us. Friends have moved away, some of us have grown closer, some farther apart. My life's ambitions have change because of that one experience that caused me to reevaluate myself. And when I finally cried when I though about Darryl, I was sad but thankful that I had taken something away from the experience.

Statement # 6

◆ This engineering student convincingly writes why he wishes to pursue a career in medicine rather than engineering

After three years of calculating, solving, estimating, and extrapolating, one conviction has remained in my mind: my main interest still lies in medicine. As an engineer I have programmed computers and designed chemical plants, but my original inclinations have not changed. I want to learn about the human body, understand the way it acts, and help those who suffer from its maladies. My decision to become a doctor is not one brought about by a process of elimination; rather, it is one that has been firmly established through the contents of my coursework and various personal experiences.

As an undergraduate chemical engineer, I have studied a variety of disciplines which I believe have done much for my abilities to analyze and solve problems in a logical and rigorous fashion. Yet, throughout my academic endeavors my premedical classes have fascinated me the most. These subjects have been my main focus and had led me to work in health-related laboratories during the summers. My first summer at M.I.T. I worked for the biology department where I evaluated the correlation between Alzheimer's disease and the loss of cells in the brainstem. This past summer I worked on a molecular analysis of mutagenesis by the liver carcinogen aflatoxin B1. Working in research laboratories showed me an aspect of science that was previously unfamiliar to me. I realized the amount of persistence required of researchers when approaching problems and came to appreciate the extent of involvement associated with scientific discoveries. But during my research I could not help but wonder how I was helping the Alzheimer's or cancer patient who could not wait for experimental results and needed immediate care. Although research is the inherent precursor of medical advances, I am more interested in its impact rather than in the actual process and would like to apply my interests in a setting that involves more human interaction.

While I realize that the desire to work with people is common to most who pursue the medical field, I cannot overemphasize my interest in listening to and helping those who are in need. As a high school student I volunteered at a hospital where my responsibilities included feeding and talking to patients. Although I was not helping them in a medical sense, they showed sincere appreciation for the time I spent with them. The patients needed as much personal attention as they did treatment, and I became more aware of that after an illness struck in my own family. From the time my mother was diagnosed with lung cancer until the time of her death, I saw the life of a patient as I had never seen before. My mother was physically and psychologically dependent on her doctors, yet their dry and unemotional prognoses were as damaging as the disease itself. I was infuriated at the stoic role they played in her treatment and promised to do things differently if ever in their position. The interplay of treatment and empathy is critical to the patient's condition, and as a physician I will try my best to achieve a favorable balance.

I have wanted to be a doctor as long as I can remember and my undergraduate experience has assured me that the decision is the right one. While my coursework has given me depth, other events and activities have given me breadth, and I feel qualified to enter the medical field. If given the opportunity, I am prepared to make a commitment to what I believe is the most intellectually and emotionally challenging career.

Statement # 7

- ◆ This student notes that as a son of a surgeon he has been exposed to medicine all of his life
- ◆ Here the student contrasts the work of the clinician to that of the researcher and decides he wants to combine the two
- ◆ He refers to his unusual background in the Israeli military which, he believes, makes him a stronger candidate

There are two types of medical doctors in the world: Those who know how to write and those who know medicine.

As a child, I would often ask my father why he was not a full-time professor at the university. In response my father, a dedicated surgeon, but only a part-time lecturer, would smile at me while defending his choice of careers. "Son," he would say, "there are two types of medical doctors in the world: Those who know how to write and those who know medicine." By the former, he sarcastically referred to physicians exclusively engaged in research and thus the writing of scientific articles. By the latter, my father referred to physicians like himself, who spend most of their time practicing clinical medicine, leaving them little or no time for research. Little did I understand back then about the inevitable trade-offs confronting my father as a physician.

Today, looking back at my four years of education at MIT, I feel as though I have completed the first step toward becoming perhaps a "third kind of physician." One who strives to simultaneously devote himself to clinical practice as well as research activities. One whose time spent in the operating room saving lives is not only his source of satisfaction, but also his motivation and inspiration for spending time in the laboratory. My father, who began practicing medicine when the state of Israel was still in its infancy, could not afford what was then perceived as the luxury of independent research, while supporting a family in an environment where mere survival was not a commodity to be taken for granted. As research opportunities for my father were scarcely in existence, his major intellectual gratification came from his ability to provide me with the best of education thanks to his uncompromising devotion to his patients and profession. I strongly believe that it is my responsibility today to use my father's gift of my training as a research scientist, and harness it to the benefit of my future patients and family with the same ardor through which he established his reputation as an exemplary surgeon.

But there is more to my aspirations than merely fulfilling my moral social obligations and facing the intellectual challenges of the fascinating world of applied science. The two are not separate entities. It is my conviction that just as my father could not have afforded to devote himself solely to medical research, the physicians of my generation cannot afford to be exclusively engaged in clinical practice without being involved, at least to some degree, in research efforts. Nevertheless, I still believe that even in today's subspecialized medicine, the medical researcher cannot afford to lose contact with the patient. After all, it is the patient whose improved quality of life ultimately defines the success or failure of any research endeavors, regardless of their intrinsic intellectual values.

I am currently completing my MIT master's thesis in the field of Materials Science and Engineering at AT&T Bell Laboratories.

Understanding matter's intrinsic and extrinsic properties and behavior is what materials science is all about. Having the ability to manipulate the physiochemical and structural characteristic parameters of matter to achieve the desired mechanical, electrical, and optical properties is what materials engineering is all about. Fascinated by the unique properties of polymeric systems and intrigued by nature's magical ability to engineer biopolymer-based tissues of incredible specificity, I have chosen to focus my future research interests in the study of high performance biomaterial applications. My experience with polymers both in academia and in the industrial laboratory environment have convinced me that indeed our knowledge and understanding of the behavior of polymer systems is key to the advancement of future biomaterials. It seems inevitable that in years to come these materials will increasingly replace damaged and aged tissues and organs of the human body. It is the implementation of biomaterial implants in today's medicine that has already saved patients from total loss of limbs. In fact, my mother was one such fortunate patient last year as her arm was close to complete amputation as a result of a car accident.

The interface between the biomaterial and the living cell on its surrounding biopolymer matrix is the interface between materials science and biology. The interaction between the biomaterial implant and the biochemical environment of the host is the interaction between the materials scientist and the physician. It is in this interface between the organic tissue material and the implanted composite biomaterial within the patient that I see my future as both researcher and clinician. The engineering of future biomaterials for medical applications and the study of the materials' behavior in vivo is a fascinating challenge to those of us who delve into the "gray" areas of this interdisciplinary field. Though it is extremely difficult for me to portray myself as an individual personality apart from my technical capabilities and interests, I find it vital to share a bit of my personal history. As a future clinician, I feel that perhaps the most important stages of my development took place during my three years of compulsory military service in the Israeli army. That period was, more than anything else, a lesson in interpersonal relationships and mutual understanding between an extremely diverse community. Through rigorous training and discipline that often stretched from sunrise to sunrise, we learned to appreciate the values of mutual support and help as a means of surviving under harsh conditions. The meaning of diversity gained yet another dimension in my perception as I became an international student in the multicultural microcosm of MIT. Equipped with some fundamental academic experience and research tools, and not less importantly with my personal background, I hoped that in spite of my being an international student, I will be considered as a potential candidate for your program.

Statement # 8

◆ The strongest point in this essay is the mentoring/ modeling role played by Dr. XXX

I was born in Korea. At the age of four, my family moved to the United States and settled in Wisconsin, where my father began a career as a civil engineer. In my youth, I was fortunate to know Dr. XXX. He visited my family often as he was a close friend of my father. When I started to decide on a future career, I consulted the wise Dr. XXX. I remember the long conversations we had. He strongly recommended the field of medicine: Charley, you can help many patients," "Charley, medicine needs bright people like your-self," and "Charley, you can meet many interesting people," he urged.

I followed his guidance. Later, as a high school and college stu-dent, my volunteer experiences reinforced Dr. XXX's notion of "meeting and helping people." I was originally introduced to com-munity service through my Catholic high school, which strongly encouraged its students to spend time in the community. My ser-vices ranges from St. Lukes' Hospital in Milwaukee to the Marga-ret Fuller House in Cambridge to a small town in Appalachia, Kentucky. Of all my experiences, I learned the most from my stay in Appalachia. After helping to build a home or visiting patients in a nursing home, my friends and I didn't receive the heaping thanks that usually awaited us from the volunteer coordinator. Rather, the Appalachians eyed us suspiciously as outsiders in the faraway town. Eventually their suspicions gave way to a natural hospitality and down home humor, for which I will always be grateful. While there are many ways for one to help others, it was my notion of helping people combined with an aptness for science that steered me to be a doctor.

In studying the premedical curriculum at MIT, I have also come to appreciate the benefits that basic science can offer the practice of medicine. If the goal of medicine is to cure disease, then under-standing how a disease works on the molecular level will guide efforts to design ways to cure them. A powerful example of scien-tific understanding leading to more effective medical treatment is immunization. Years ago, children were immunized from small-pox, and all, or nearly all, of those children never suffered from that disease. Although *to cure* is often thought of in the context of restoring a sick person to health, I believe that treatments, like vaccines, which preempt the onset of symptoms, are a more potent method of *curing*. With the growing technology to study the way diseases work, I am interested in researching new methods and drugs to cure them. In training to be a physician-scientist, I am applying as a M.D./Ph.D. candidate.

For the last two years, I have been a member of Dr. YYY's group at the Whitehead Institute for Biomedical Research, where I have studied the protein-folding problem. My interest in protein-folding was initially sparked by the prospect of *de novo* protein design for therapy. My project centered around the use of limited proteolysis to separate independently folded domains of proteins. Through biochemical methods, I have managed to isolate three pieces of one protein which together form an eight-stranded beta-barreled structure. Currently, I am studying this unique system with circular dichroism and nuclear magnetic resonance. Working with as bright a group as Dr. YYY's and being able to follow the advances in biomedical research has incited my conviction that training in both medicine and science is valuable.

Statement # 9

♦ Very engaging opening quotations
♦ Though the theme of death is unusual for a personal statement, it is effective here

"What do I write about?" I asked a fellow premed.

"That's a stupid question. Write about how helpless you felt when your grandmother died and how the experience motivated you to become a doctor, of course."

"But nobody close to me has died or even been seriously sick."

My friend just looked at me sympathetically and said, "Good luck getting into med. school, buddy."

Well, I'm not a good liar so I'll just have to go with the less sensational truth. My first motivations for becoming a doctor came when I was 12 years old and was, at the time, very much afraid of dying. Every night, as I lay in bed trying to fall asleep, I thought about death. "I don't want to die," I would say to myself repeatedly until the gurgling of my fish tank and the rumbling of trucks on the distant highway mercifully ushered in sleep.

Around the time I was obsessed with death, I developed a fascination for biology. Biology had the power to dissect complex life forms into something almost mechanical. People were simply ordered collections of unconscious cells performing programmed tasks. To "cure" aging, I thought, "I'll just figure out which cells are malfunctioning and fix them." Filled with childish self-confidence, I resolved to become a doctor and find a cure before someone else beat me to it.

During the summers after my sophomore and junior years of high school, I worked as an intern in a biomedical research laboratory. I investigated actin-myosin interaction in smooth muscle tissue. Although I didn't fully understand the science behind my experiments, I nevertheless felt important. I realized that even my seemingly trite experiments were somehow contributing to the better understanding of the human body. My initial exposure to research triggered in me the impulse to experiment, to do things that no one else has ever done. For the first time, I tasted the thrill of making a discovery and more frequently, felt the heavy frustration of failing time after time.

Eager to learn more biology and continue performing research en route to my self-ordained crusade to conquer death, I entered the Massachusetts Institute of Technology. Shortly after I started school, however, I lost my obsession for death. Maybe it was the busy social life or the sleepless nights spent studying instead of lying in bed counting the years, days, and hours I have left to live. Whatever the reason, my studies lost their original focus. Instead, I found myself driven by my original interest in biology. While my physics and calculus books were instant remedies for insomnia, my biology texts read like good fiction. Although the biology I have learned has been primarily cellular and molecular, I don't feel that I am looking at life through too narrow an aperture. Only through the elucidation of the workings of single cells can the functioning of entire organisms be understood.

For the past two years, I have been conducting research on determinants of cellular shape and motility under Professor ZZZ at the Important Research Center. Currently, I am studying a gene encoding protein involved in neurite extension. Although I enjoy my time in the lab, performing research is a contest test of my character. Every day, I wage a battle against frustration. Yet, even though I dread coming to lab each morning to face failure, the minute chance of success always drags me in. The ecstasy of achieving positive results I first felt five years ago has been magnified. Understanding the biology behind the gels and the columns and being able to read journal articles and critique their authors as a colleague is a glorious feeling.

I am excited by research that leads to a means to rescue or preserve the human body. Clinical applications can potentially be found for nearly all biology research; I want to be someone that makes the connection. I realize though that patients are not mere potential research subjects; they are human beings whose lives depend on the talents of doctors. I am sure, as I prepare to unite test tube with stethoscope, that the piquancy and sense of fulfillment that I have gotten from research will only intensify when people's lives, not journal publication, hinge on my results.

Statement # 10

- The opening paragraph, which conveys a personal experience, draws the reader's attention
- Throughout the essay the author draws on personal experiences to show that she would be an excellent candidate

I suppose the first time I ever wanted to be a doctor, was when my mother had cancer. I didn't cry when I first heard the news; I didn't understand. It wasn't until I realized that my mom was in pain from the tumors that I cried. That was about a month before her surgery. I was suddenly irrationally tiptoeing around in fear of doing something wrong since I thought that God might take away my mom or cause her more pain if I did anything bad. I was terrified that if I told anyone how scared I was or if I wasn't completely good, I would lose her. For the space of about two weeks, I couldn't eat or sleep very well and I clung to mom when she was home. On her last visit to her oncologist before the surgery, my entire family went for the consultation. My mother was having difficulty walking due to the pain and I couldn't stand to watch. I ran across the hall from the reception area and hid in the corner of a blue carpeted room. I found out later that it was my mom's doctor's office.

I think the first inklings of trust for medical science started when my mom's oncologist found me. I remember a grand fatherly look-ing man in a white coat sat me down and wiped my wet face. He talked to me for a few minutes but in that space of time, he broke down the superstitious barriers that I had been clinging to. Cancer, he said, happens to many people. And it doesn't happen because they had done something wrong in their life. He said he could prove that and I believed him. He then said he was going to try and help my mom get better and explained that it would require surgery to remove the tumors. I was still scared that my mom was going to die but at least at that time, I finally accepted that it was all right to be scared. After the surgery was successful and my mother recov-ered, I became extremely interested in medicine and biology. I was amazed that another person could change someone else's life in such a great way.

Over the next few years, my hobby was reading about infectious diseases, clinical treatments, and "miracle story" cures. I bought about a hundred books with my allowance money on anything medically or biologically (gross anatomy) related and my parents gave me all the encouragement. They relented without any com-plaints (even on school nights) when I would confiscate the living room TV during a show that had anything to do with biological science; and they also understood when I brought stray animals home with crude bandages wrapped around them. I considered becoming a veterinarian, but being highly allergic to long-haired cats quickly changed my mind. My parents also forbade us to have four-legged pets when my brother's science fair project (20 rats being fed different diets of carbohydrates and fats) escaped from their cages and roamed the house for a week until their capture. Without any animal patients (aside from birds and fish which you really can't play with), I wisely decided I should look at a medical career with humans instead.

When I entered college, I had a rather naive perspective toward the field of medicine. It was too unidimensional and flawless in nature. I wasn't completely sure that it was what I wanted to do for a lifetime. I spent two summers as a volunteer intern in the Human Monoclonal Antibody lab at New England Deaconess Hospital. The lab researched antibodies to HIV and T-cell specific virus. It was an incredible academic experience from the side of research but I also learned what medicine is really like. My supervisor, Dr. XXX, was an oncologist. All of his patients were terminally ill, some from cancer and others from AIDS. At first, I internally balked at the sight of some of his patients. Most exhibited the ravages of skin cancers, brain tumors, and immune system shut downs. But soon, I was able to completely view his patients from two perspectives: the first being from a purely physical/scientific slant and the second from a normal human relations perspective.

The first summer I was there, I did not have very much contact with the patients. I spent most of my time in the lab. The second summer, after my uncle and cousin died, I asked to go around on all of Dr. XXX's rounds at the hospital. He agreed and I escorted him when he examined his patients. I realized then how emotionally draining yet inspirational the rounds can be. I became aware of the importance of the patient's perspective of his/her physician and how it effects his/her subsequent behavior and recovery. Doctors are fallible and with their imperfections, they can be either too humane or entirely inhumane. I learned that there exists a thin line between being in empathy with one's patient and yet maintaining the detachment necessary for an authority figure.

Perhaps it was from feeling of guilt or sadness over the death in my family that made me initially so intensely interested in the patients' welfare, but I soon continued meeting with the patients because I wanted to know whether they were making progress in their treatments or not. I spent many hours talking to patients who were in the midst of chemotherapy treatments or recovering from surgery. These people inspired me to live my life fully and completely because they continued to do so despite their illnesses and pain. My perspective toward life became enriched that summer because I realized just what things in life were most important to me. I knew by the end of the summer that my future career would need some interaction with helping people. Helping people to change their lives for the better brings joy into my own life.

From then on, plans for my future career were solely a matter of logistics and filling in blank spots. I chose to pursue a medical degree with the intent to continue in public service along the national level. I believe that I will be able to achieve these goals because I plan to apply myself completely to these pursuits. Ultimately, however, I want to be an excellent doctor who will be seen by patients as a humanist sincerely concerned about their welfare.

I know I have so much to learn and train for but I feel strongly that if given the opportunity, I could do it or devote my life to trying.

Statement # 11

♦ Using family, fraternity, the military, and research — all traditional values — this successful applicant developed an interesting personal statement

Many experiences have shaped my life. They have all taught me lessons and contributed to the set of ideals I possess and the goals I wish to attain. I have depended on these to guide me in making decisions which bring into focus things that I value the most. Among the more influential contributors to my experiences are my family, my fraternity, Army ROTC, and my research.

Some of the most important things I've learned from my parents are to respect and care for others. My mothers works in a nursing home as a housekeeper. Not only does she do her job, but she also cares for all the people she meets. She is interested in their lives and spends time talking to them while working. I see the effect my mother has on these elderly people. When my mother enters the room they smile because they know she cares. My mother also does little extra things for them such as baking them cookies and bringing our cat in for them to play with. She also visits them on days when she doesn't have to work. Her selfless acts have motivated me to pursue a career which will benefit others. This is one of the reasons why I want to become a doctor.

In addition, my parents urged me to set my own standards of excellence and to live up to my potential. I can always remember the support my father gave me when I was involved in tennis. He would rejoice whenever I won, and more importantly, he would tell me to pick my head up when I lost. When I was a junior in high school, my tennis team missed the regional conference playoffs by one game. I knew I could have won my match, but my lack of self confidence prevented me from turning the match around when I started to fall behind. After the match, my father told me to set my goals and work hard. From that point, I worked on different aspects of the game, and by the end of the summer, I felt more confident in my game and my abilities. The following year my team made the playoffs for the first time in seven years.

Entering M.I.T. was a frightening experience for me as it was for most of my classmates. However, in the first few days, I joined Kappa Sigma Fraternity and was surrounded by friends who were willing to help me with any problems. One thing that remains in my mind is the help I received from our house tutor. At first, the life at M.I.T. seemed hard to handle. Difficult problem sets and papers were due each week along with lengthy reading assignments.

My workload seemed unbearable until the house tutor sat down with me. He showed me how to plan and organize my work more efficiently, and more importantly, how to prioritize my assignments. Before, I wasted time on esoteric concepts or got stuck on small details. Now I focus on understanding the concepts and then use them to grasp the details. Today I give back what I had received when I was a freshman. I volunteer my time to tutor students in organic chemistry. I feel proud helping these students, and I can relate to them; I was once in their place. Tutoring has helped me feel comfortable getting my point across to others.

Army ROTC has had a profound effect on my life. The program has strengthened my discipline and leadership skills. Every two weeks cadets change leadership positions from platoon leader down to team leader in their class level. Through these positions, I have gained many skills such as how to march a platoon and how to assert myself, taking charge when I was the leader. I have also learned to respect the decisions of others in leadership positions when I was not. Army ROTC has shown me how to give my best at everything I do. An example of this can be seen in the ranger challenge competition. The M.I.T. ranger challenge team consists of the best cadets from our school who compete in a three-day contest against other teams in the brigade. The competition consists of seven events that test physical endurance as well as individual skills and knowledge. I have been on the team for two years, and next fall I will be the captain. There were times in the competition, such as during the 10K ruck march, when I felt like giving up. But when this happened, my teammates encouraged me and forced me to push myself to my limits. I discovered that my limits were more than I thought, and if I push myself, I can achieve what I never thought was possible.

During my college years, I have had the opportunity to do research in different labs under top quality professors. For my first research project, I worked for Dr. XXX in the M.I.T. Chemistry Department on the synthesis of isomalabaricane, an antitumor drug. In order to set the correct ring backbone of the molecule, my advisor suggested I use an enzyme in yeast that catalyzes a similar reaction. His ability to apply his knowledge has inspired me to learn more, so that someday I might be able to do the same. Last summer, I worked for Dr. YYY in the U.C. Irvine Chemistry Department. I generalized an addition reaction to make three substituted glutarates by using cuprate chemistry. This summer, I am working on the characterization of SRCR domains on macrophage scavenger receptors under Dr. ZZZ in the M.I.T. Biology Department. I will determine what classes of ligands bind to the receptor domain. Next, I will determine how many ligands it binds by performing radioimmunoassays on a system in which the receptor domain is expressed on mammalian cell surfaces. During medical school, I hope to further develop my interests in research either part time or as a Ph.D./M.D. student.

Extracurricular activities help me to relax. I am a brother in Alpha Chi Sigma, a chemistry service fraternity. Every year brothers take turns teaching a chemistry-oriented class to interested third and sixth graders. Brothers also participate in Boy Scout Day in which we help Boy Scouts receive their chemistry merit badges. Other ways that I spend my free time include competing in sports such as ultimate frisbee, hockey, and softball. I have wanted to become a doctor for a long time. The experiences that I have gone though have given me numerous skills and have made me the person that I am today. I am confident, motivated, and resourceful. I listen to the opinions of others and I am not afraid to change my own views in light of what is said. I feel that throughout my life I have gained and refined the skills necessary to succeed in medical school and become a skillful, compassionate doctor.

Statement # 12

- ◆ This applicant declares and then proves that she has the attributes important for a medical student
- ◆ She demonstrates a lifelong interest in medicine and pediatrics
- ◆ Using effective examples, she builds a powerful case for admission to a top medical school — a goal which she ultimately reached

I feel that I have all qualities necessary to be a successful medical student — I enjoy science, care about people, and am not afraid of hard work. Please consider me an eager future medical student.

Ever since elementary school, I have wanted to be a doctor and have sought opportunities to be exposed to physicians and medicine. In grade school, I collected stickers like all my fellow female students. However, I collected the stickers with the goals of giving them to future patients whom I hoped would enjoy them as much as I did then. While volunteering at San Jose Medical Center, I worked in the Emergency Room and saw a blood stained man with stab wounds. Doctors, nurses, and technicians worked together as a team while some patients were forgotten in the overcrowded ER area. As an outside observer, I had the unique opportunity to see health care from both the doctor's side administering the treatment and the patient's side receiving treatment. Serving as a volunteer Spanish interpreter at the Massachusetts General Hospital, I observed the bedside manners of many caring doctors in different fields of medicine from gynecology to radiology.

Whenever I visit the doctor, I ask what the doctor is doing and why — because I am very curious and I want to learn. When working for the Dana Farber Center Institute, I stayed in a medical school dormitory and befriended the students there. I asked them about medical school and took note of their life-style, knowing someday I would also be a medical student. Needing to isolate T-cells while working at Stanford, I learned to draw blood. At first, I was scared and repulsed by drawing blood. However, when I thought of venipuncture from a scientist's viewpoint and was interested in the way veins swell when tied at the upper arm, my fear and aversion disappeared. I have enjoyed everything I have observed relating to medicine from physiology to how to give a physical examination, and I am eager to learn more.

From these scientific observations and conversations, I learned that it is very difficult and yet very important to educate people about their own bodies. While working with the Women's Health Education Network (WHEN) doing our Contraceptive Road Show, I learned how to phrase answers to questions from individuals with diverse backgrounds. A challenge in medicine, which I am ready to embrace, is to be able to communicate with patients of all background, ages, and states of health.

Having been exposed to the bloody and demanding side of medicine as well, I am still interested in becoming a doctor and feel that this is the field for me. I have seen the zombie-like third year medical students tired from being on call and I am willing to become a zombie if that is what it takes to be the best doctor I can be for my future patients.

My goal has always been to become a doctor, but I realize now that my goal has expanded as I have grown older. I am no longer content with simply becoming a M.D. From experiences with my doctor-uncle and my advisor, I learned that I want to be more — I want to be a caring and patient doctor.

My premed advisor taught me that each patient is not a case but a relationship to be developed. If the patient does not trust you, he will not come back and then you cannot help him. Meeting new people is always an exciting experience for me, because each new person is like another story. Everyone has something special about them and if you are patient, you can find each person's special quality if you talk to him. As a sorority member, a class officer, and a student, I have developed many relationships and hopefully, I have also built trust between others and myself.

I will strive to be a humanistic doctor. My uncle once told me never to forget that it is important to make the patient not only physically better but also mentally better. By that, he meant the patient must *feel* well. A doctor cannot always cure, but she can always comfort. I once had a corneal ulcer and although the doctor who first saw me could not help me because he was not a specialist, he could comfort me and he did. When he sat down, placed his hand on my shoulder, and told me that everything was going to be

OK, he projected an aura of calm and caring which made me feel less scared and less worried. It amazed me what a simple touch and kind word could do. I hope to become such a doctor.

Statement #13

♦ This student effectively explains her decision, late in her college career, to become a physician

I can think of no profession more satisfying than being a doctor. I have considered the options, and unlike some who all their lives want only to be a doctor, the path I have taken to share this conviction has been circuitous and long. But it is not a path I regret. It has allowed me to discover the spectrum of my capabilities and decide what I truly aspire for in life. I want to face every day of my career knowing that I will be directly affecting someone's life. I want to know that my work will make the quality of a person's life better, that I will be helping to keep families together, and that people will come to me when in need. Yes, there are other professions that will allow me these opportunities, but I can think of no better way than to become a physician.

I have come to a point in my life that I am able to assess my strengths and, rather than just settle into a career owing to my capabilities, discover what truly drives me. At MIT I have had the opportunity to fully realize my skills as an engineer. I have been mentored by people renowned in their fields of study and have learned in an environment of healthy, yet intense, competition. I have worked in research and felt the excitement of proving a hypothesis or completing a design. I am proud of my accomplishments and have no doubts as to my abilities as an engineer. But, I also realize my most valuable skill is not one that can be taught or learned through a book; it is that of dealing with people and arises only from a desire to care, listen, and respond to those in need.

I have worked extensively in peer counseling and felt the overwhelming sense of content that arises only when you know you have reached out and helped someone, whether a stranger or friend. Such a feeling will always surpass the impersonal sense of accomplishment that work in research or industry, for me, seem to provide. Some may think me an idealist, but I know I have faced disappointment and hence do not delude myself about the glory of medicine. I have felt the helplessness of seeing someone in need sink deeper into their despair, beyond my reach, as I am left to standby, powerless. As a physician I will undoubtedly face such disappointments, but with such a high stake as life itself, the times of success will make medicine worth the struggle.

I have also seen my father as a doctor. But, it is more his role as a patient that has shaped my attitude toward medicine. My earliest experience in a hospital was visiting him after his first heart attack. Over the years that followed, I learned of his diabetes and watched him take insulin. I also learned of the partnership my family formed with his physician to save my father from his ill health. Although he suffered a fatal heart attack seven years later, my family will always be grateful for the care and prolonged life that this man, a doctor, helped provide.

Death is inevitable. This reality is something I have had to understand and accept since then. As a physician I will not be able to promise miracles, but I will have the resources to help make them possible. If I can help return a husband to his wife, a mother to her child, then I will have accomplished my goals of facing each day knowing that I am positively affecting a life.

For me, being an engineer has meant employing technology to improve the quality of life by overcoming human limitations. Medicine takes this opportunity to its limits — it is about saving lives by battling with our most formidable limitation yet — the inevitability of death. I find this challenge irresistible. I realize that there is so much I do not know, so many challenges I cannot even fathom. But I do know that there is nothing I want more from life than to be given this opportunity to best utilize my skills — as a doctor.

Statement # 14

◆ Though a different style of writing from the previous essays, this student also explains a career change to a premedical course of studies

What in the world am I doing here?
It was the summer before my senior year at MIT. I was sitting at my desk at Lincoln Laboratories designing tests to measure thermodynamic emissions in a space simulated environment. When I was first accepted into the Engineering Internship Program with Lincoln Labs, I was thrilled to finally apply what I learned in my engineering courses. Moreover, I had wanted to work in space technology ever since I was a young child dreaming of becoming an astronaut. Yet, there I was at my desk, wondering why I felt unfulfilled. Although engineering would always pique my curiosity and academic interests, I desired a career that would have a more personal and direct impact on people. I began to realize that a career in *medicine* would allow me to help improve people's lives while providing me with a lifetime of fascinating discoveries.

But do I have what it takes?
Incredible mental and physical stamina are "prerequisites" for an avionics major at MIT, as it combines aeronautical with electrical engineering. However, there are many stimulating course

projects which make the many "all-nighters" worthwhile. For example, in Space Systems Engineering, I helped to design the life support system in a class effort to propose a viable rescue vehicle for the Space Shuttle astronauts. Our research culminated in a final report and presentation of the vehicle design to NASA and industry officials. Classes such as this have developed my capability to perform and work with others under extreme pressures and have particularly honed my skills in thinking and problem solving.

As the captain and starting quarterback of both my high school and college varsity football teams, the ability to perform under pressure was absolutely essential. As a leader on the MIT team, I struggled not only to fight back from injuries, but also to motivate a perennially losing team. Leading by example and fostering respect amongst the players, I helped to arouse a sense of team pride and dedication to win. In my final season in 1993, MIT football earned a trip to the league championship and I received the "Special Contributions" award from the coaches of the league for outstanding team leadership. Having played for over ten years, football was more than just a sport to me; it has developed much of my character, determination, and work ethic that has driven me to excel in all that I do.

Most importantly, I feel I have always had a great compassion for people, which I attribute to my mother. As an RN for most of her life, she raised me to be charitable to those less fortunate through service. As a volunteer in the emergency ward at the Massachusetts General Hospital in Boston, I helped to comfort and transport newly admitted patients. Having been through several operations and much physical therapy myself, I understand how it feels to be a frightened and worried patient. Therefore, I knew that a friendly hello, holding a hand, or any gesture to show that someone genuinely cared, could make a difference in how a patient felt and even affect their progress. Along the same lines, I have also particularly enjoyed trying to make a difference in the lives of children. Whether it has been coordinating big brother events for Cambridge inner city youths, organizing walk-a-thons for abused children, or even teaching bible study to first graders, helping children has always been a source of tremendous joy and fulfillment.

After much reflection upon these and other experiences, I felt that I had the stamina, drive and compassion needed to pursue a career as a physician. Thus, at the start of my senior year, I drove to my premed classes with zeal and began work on a biochemical study to reduce cholesterol using rabbits at MIT's Langer Laboratory. After graduating in December of 1993, I moved back home to New York City in order to work and help with my family's financial difficulties. However, I also wanted to take advantage of the time to explore medicine more fully.

My love for children led me to the Pediatric Hematology/Oncology division of Columbia Presbyterian Hospital, where I have been working since the winter of this year. I am currently involved in a molecular biological study, characterizing mutations in the ferrochelatase gene of children suffering from erythropoietic protoporphyria. In addition to learning the methods involved in the isolation and cloning of DNA, it has been especially motivating to know that my work is contributing to the search for a cure for those afflicted with this disease.

Also, on a part-time basis in the same division, I have been working closely with doctors and nurses in the data management of children's cancer therapies. The patients I work around, some newborn, are afflicted with cancers ranging from acute lymphoblastic leukemia to Wilms' Tumor. A couple of the children I play with are even terminally ill. It is such a tragic and helpless feeling, yet the doctors and nurses I look up to never cease their efforts to increase the quality of their patients' lives. I have faced the harsh reality that, although my stamina, drive and compassion may help many in the future, there may also be many heartbreaking disappointments.

From my learning experiences, I am confident and excited about my decision to pursue a career in medicine. I feel that I have the character and the potential to provide people with the best possible healthcare. I look forward to the many challenges and new discoveries that lie ahead.

Chapter Seven
. . . .

THE INTERVIEW

More than 99 percent of U.S. medical schools require their serious applicants to have interviews. Thus, if you are a good candidate there is a strong probability that you will be interviewed.

Most interviewing takes place at the medical school and includes two separate interviews and a tour of the medical school. A few medical schools, such as Harvard Medical School, schedule interviews in distant locations to spare students the expense and inconvenience of travel. This is the exception. Budget time and money to travel to the medical schools. You need to know far more about where you may spend the next four years. If, by chance, you were admitted following regional interviews and you did not visit schools, you should, at the very least, visit the school you plan to attend.

Honesty in an interview
. . . .
is made up of three
. . . .
elements — truth,
. . . .
consistency, and candor.

H. Anthony Medley

Typically, one of the interviews is conducted by a member of the admissions committee and the other is arranged with another member of the faculty or staff. The tour is often led by a student. Interviews with multiple students and one interviewer or multiple interviewers and one student are less common.

According to Janine C. Edwards, Ph.D., Director, Research in Medical Education and Associate Professor, Department of Surgery, St. Louis University School of Medicine, *et. al.*, there are several reasons for the medical school interview. First, they help gather factual data and clarify details on the applicant's file. In addition, they provide more information on nonintellectual characteristics such as motivation, leadership, altruism, and interpersonal skills that may not necessarily be available from other sources. Moreover, the interview supplements the material presented on the primary and secondary applications, thereby aiding the schools in the overall decision-making process, and serves as an opportunity to verify application materials. Finally, when top or prime candidates are identified, the interviewer may attempt to recruit those who are found to have the personality and ethical qualities to become good physicians.

A small number of medical schools include interviews with specially trained psychiatrists who attempt to identify candidates with abnormal personality disorders. Such identification may be important in the admission decision process.

At approximately 85 percent of the schools, the interview format includes a one-to-one meeting between an interviewer and an applicant. A minority of schools have group interviews, panels, or combinations of various formats. One hundred percent of the schools include faculty and staff in the interview process, and 72 percent of the schools also involve students in the interview and tour. Thirty-four percent of the schools report that alumni are part of the process. Eighty percent of the schools say that at least one member of the admissions committee participates in the interview of every candidate. Forty-six percent of the schools require two interviews. Twenty-nine percent want only one separate interview. Fourteen percent schedule three separate interviews during an applicant's visit. Four interviews are required by one percent of the schools. And nine percent had no limit on the number of interviews.

Medical school application interviews may be classified as structured, semi-structured, and unstructured. Structured interviews generally involve asking all applicants certain standard questions. (Fifty percent of the schools said that they had such standard questions.) Usually, there are only a limited number of interviewers, often between two and five. Such limiting of interviewers is believed to improve reliability. Semistructured interviews have some of these criterion, and unstructured interviews have none.

James B. Puryear, Ph.D., the Director of Student Affairs and Secretary of the Medical School Admissions Committee, Medical College of Georgia, Augusta, *et. al.*, asked 107 medical schools to rank — on a scale of one to four — the order and importance of the GPA, MCAT scores, references, and interview in the selection of applicants. Fifty-eight schools, or 54 percent of those responding, listed the interview as the most significant criterion in the selection of students. When evaluating this statistic, however, it is crucial to note that much of the selection process occurs before a student is ever asked for an interview. In some schools, as many as

90 percent of the applicants are screened out before the top ten percent are selected for an interview.

It is the interviewing policy of some schools to de-emphasize academic performance and focus on nonacademic issues. This apparently leads to the selection of more students with high ratings in leadership, range of interests, and motivation.

Stephen R. Smith, M.D., M.P.H., Associate Dean of Medicine and Professor of Family Medicine, Brown University Program in Medicine, evaluated the medical school and residency performances of students admitted with and without an admission interview. He compared the grades of distinction and grades of deficiency in the preclinical and clinical courses of 113 students admitted between 1983 and 1985 without an interview and 67 students admitted from 1980 to 1982 with an interview. He also noted the scores on the National Boards Part I and Part II and studied evaluation scores from residency program directors. It is interesting to observe that Smith found no significant differences between the group that was admitted with an interview and the group that was admitted without an interview.

Let the world know you are as you are not as you think you should be, because sooner or later, if you are posing, you will forget the pose, and then where are you?

Fanny Brice

At the 1994 Annual Meeting of the Association of American Medical Colleges, Carol Elam, Ed.D., an Assistant Dean for Admission at the University of Kentucky College of Medicine, *et. al.,* shared the results of her analysis of 950 interview reports written on 465 matriculants at the University of Kentucky College of Medicine during the years 1984–1988. Seventy-seven interviewers were involved in the study, and the reports, which ranged in length from 15 to 632 words differed dramatically from one another. "Perhaps the most striking finding is the general lack of comparability of recorded material across interviewers," Dr. Elam wrote. "Some interviewers include much information, others made one-word judgments." Dr. Elam said that the written reports revealed that the University of Kentucky College of Medicine considers certain attributes, such as experience and knowledge of the profession, of particular importance. Less significance was placed on the applicant's performance in medical research or background in ancillary settings.

Dr. Elam found that interviewers wrote about the applicants' sources of motivation and commented on their dedication and caring. They also discussed their ability to interact in a group. Consequently, people-oriented applicants who work well with others may have a significant advantage over shy or quiet applicants. Being confident and articulate was felt to be a positive attribute.

Dr. Elam said that applicants who described a support system of family and peers, positive work experiences, and the ability to organize commitments and delay gratification, showed a well-developed sense of responsibility. Knowing how to overcome adversity and maximize available opportunities were also deemed valued attributes.

Practice Pointers for Interviews

Some of these suggestions were derived from Sweaty Palms: The Neglected Art of Being Interviewed *by Anthony Medley.*

If you are old enough and smart enough to be applying to medical school, you may think some of these suggestions are simply silly. It is, you may mumble, a waste of your time to read them. But you never can tell. Some small seemingly insignificant action on your part could make the difference. So sit back and read carefully.

First and foremost, be certain of the time and place of the interview and the name(s) of the interviewer(s). Arrive a few minutes early. Never be late. Bring a pen and a notebook. Remember the interviewer's name. Do not chew gum. Do not sit down until the interviewer sits or asks you to seat yourself. During the interview process, it will be your responsibility to sell yourself as a potential medical student. You must have an honest presentation. You must make the interviewer feel good about you.

Take time to prepare for the interview. Before each interview read all the materials mailed from the school. You should be aware of the course curriculum, research opportunities, clinical settings, and internship placements. Have some questions to ask about these four areas or other areas of particular interest to you. Prepare answers to commonly asked questions such as those on Table 7-1. Know how you will respond to any problems with your application such as why you received a low grade in a particular subject or test. And be able to describe your work and extracurricular activities.

Table 7-1
Questions You Should be Prepared to Answer

1. Why do you want to enter medicine?

2. What type of public service have you performed?

3. Tell me about your research.

4. Have you worked in a hospital? If so, describe your experience.

5. What are your career goals?

6. Why are you applying to this school?

7. What positions of leadership have you held? Describe them.

8. What did you do last summer?

9. Are any of your family members in medicine?

10. What are your career plans if you are not accepted to medical school?

Remember the interview is a time to sell yourself. Do not appear shy or withdrawn. Appear enthusiastic and articulate. When answering questions, do not be short or long winded. Maintain a positive attitude with no chips on your shoulders, even if this school is your last choice. You never can tell. It may be your only choice.

Listen to each question and think carefully before answering. Be aware of skeletons in your closet. If these do come up, be honest and objective. And definitely think positively.

Dress conservatively but comfortable. Your clothes should be clean. Pay special attention to nails and hair. Give a fresh appearance. An experienced medical school interviewer commented that women seemed be more comfortably dressed than the men. In fact, the men appeared, and probably felt more uncomfortable, especially, their interviewer noted, in their new suits and black shoes.

When I was interviewing for medical school in the late 1960s, there were applicants who spoke of stress interviews at certain prestigious medical schools. Examples included the interviewer who asked applicants to open a window that was nailed shut. The interviewer would then note how the applicant reacted to stress.

Fortunately, I never had such an interview. Nevertheless, stress could be triggered by such subtle behaviors as an interviewer's extended period of silence. It has been suggested that you do not break the silence unless you are asked to respond to a question.

Finally, there are certain things you must *not* do. Do not be arrogant or cocky. Do not show a lack of interest. Do not be a poor communicator or have poor eye contact. Do not be cold, overconfident, or dishonest. Do not give shallow answers to questions. Do not be unprepared. And do not appear unprofessional.

Try to control your nervousness. You have already passed several levels of screening. Only a minority of applicants are asked for interviews. In many schools, the majority of applicants have already been weeded out. You should feel elated that you have been selected for this final group of serious applicants. Your academic record, your MCAT scores, and letters of recommendation have spoken for themselves. The interview gives you the opportunity to show that you are an outstanding candidate who should be awarded a place in the incoming medical school class. Good Luck.

References — Chapter Seven

1. Edwards, J.C., Johnson, E.K., Molidor, J.B., "The Interview in the Admission Process," *Academic Medicine,* 65:167–176, 1990.
2. Puryear, J.B., Lewis, L.A., "Description of the Interview Process in Selecting Students for Admission to U.S. Medical Schools," *Journal of Medical Education,* 56:881–885, 1981.
3. Smith, S.R., "Medical School and Residency Performances of Students Admitted With and Without an Admission Interview," *Academic Medicine,* 66:474–476, 1991.
4. Elam, C.L., Johnson, M.M.S., Wiese, H.J., Studts, J.L., Rosenbaum, M., "Admission Interview Reports: A Content Analysis of Interviewer Comments," *Academic Medicine,* 69:563–565, 1994. Also presented by Dr. Elam at the 1994 Annual Meeting of the Association of American Medical Colleges in Boston.
5. Medley, H.A., *Sweaty Palms,* Ten Speed Press, Berkeley, California, 1992.

Chapter Eight
. . . .

MINORITY STUDENTS

For generations, the vast majority of medical schools had few if any minority students. Most were filled with white males from affluent or at least financially comfortable families. Thinking back, when I was a student, I can remember less than a handful of minority students at Georgetown.

During the late 1960s, the situation began to change. Medical schools took a proactive role to increase the enrollment of underrepresented minorities. For the first time in the history of medical education, medical schools reached out to Black Americans, American Indians, Mexican Americans, and Mainland Puerto Ricans and encouraged them to apply.

By the academic year 1994–95, of the 67,072 students attending U.S. medical schools, 7,615 or 11.4 percent were underrepresented minorities. During that same year, there were 2,288 underrepresented minority first-year new entrants. Of these, 1,519 were Black Americans, 131 were American Indians or Alaskan Native, 501 were Mexican American or Chicano, and 137 were Mainland Puerto Rican.

The impetus for change began in 1969 when the Association of American Medical Colleges (AAMC) created the Task Force on Minority Students. From 1969–1979, the enrollment of underrepresented minorities grew from 3.12 percent in 1969 to 8.0 percent in 1979. To add even more momentum to the effort, in November 1991, the AAMC developed Project 3000 by 2000 — an effort to increase the annual number of underrepresented minority first-year matriculants to 3000 by the year 2000. Project 3000 by 2000 also works to create partnerships between academic medical centers, undergraduate colleges, and local school

> *I have a dream that one day every valley shall be exalted, every hill and mountain shall be made low, the rough places will be made plains and the crooked places will be made straight . . .*
>
> **Martin Luther King Jr.**
> **August 28, 1963**

systems. Most medical schools have a local official who coordinates the program.

As a result, a large percentage of medical schools now offer outreach programs to underrepresented minorities. Eighty-seven schools have programs for high schoolers. For example, the Brown University School of Medicine Access to Medical Careers (MEDAC) identifies potential candidates while they are still in middle school. Then, just as students are about to begin high school, they are enrolled. During the summer before the tenth grade, students participate in a six-week program in which they study biology, chemistry, physics, mathematics, and communication skills. That is followed by a longitudinal program in which students have mentors and receive instruction and counseling. Those who succeed are admitted to Brown's Program in Liberal Medical Education (PLME), an eight-year combined undergraduate and medical school program, or to the Early Identification Program at one of the schools that collaborate with Brown.

Another 88 programs concentrate on students who are in college. The University of Massachusetts Medical School offers a summer enrichment opportunity for premedical students who have completed their sophomore year of college. The program has several aims, including familiarizing students with the medical school environment and improving study skills and MCAT performance. Minority or economically disadvantaged students are actively recruited. Free housing and a stipend are included.

There are also 82 programs for students who have already been accepted to medical school. Through the Office of Recruitment and Multicultural Affairs, Harvard Medical School sponsors a prematriculation summer program for minority or economically disadvantaged students who have been admitted to Harvard Medical or Harvard Dental Schools. The goal of the program is to nurture future faculty members. For eight weeks, students are assigned to laboratories at Harvard Medical School, MIT, or affiliated hospitals.

The Prematriculation Summer Program at Tufts University School of Medicine presents an extensive four-week introduction to first-year medical school courses. Classes are taught by medical school faculty, graduate students, and medical school students. There are also a wide variety of supplementary sessions and opportunities to meet with key members of the medical school staff. To further ease the transition, upper-class students are matched with incoming students.

Ten U.S. medical schools offer programs for students accepted to any medical school. The University of Virginia School of Medicine has a program that includes sections on biochemistry, cell physiology, genetics, gross anatomy, introduction to clinical medicine, and structure and function. There is even instruction in academic strategies such as improving study skills and test taking. Students conduct research, learn to make clinical observations, and receive personal counseling. For qualified minorities, stipends and travel assistance are available.

Twenty-eight medical schools offer postbaccalaureate programs at the medical school or undergraduate campus. The Morehouse School of Medicine has a five-week summer program for postbaccalaureate students including coursework in time management, biochemistry, epidemiology, histology, biochemistry, test taking, and study skills. This program is similar to the first-year medical school curriculum.

Al Hesser, Ed.D., Assistant Professor of Medical Education, Office of Minority Affairs, and Associate Director, Student Educational Enrichment Programs, and Lloyd Lewis, Ph.D., Professor of Medical Education, Curriculum Office, both at the Medical College of Georgia School of Medicine, reviewed the successes of the four-week Summer Prematriculation Program (SPP) for blacks and other nontraditional students. The study, which was conducted at the Medical College of Georgia School of Medicine, compared achievement and retention of 115 first-year medical students who participated in SPP from 1980–89 to 89 first-year students who did not participate. The SPP included coursework in most of the first-year medical school courses. While no statistically significant achievement or retention differences were observed between the two groups, the authors still believe that the SPP is an important and valuable experience. More than 90 percent of the attendees noted that the program had contributed in a positive way to their medical school adjustment.

To assist those minority students who wish to identify themselves to the medical schools, the AAMC developed the Medical Minority Applicant Registry (Med-MAR). Med-MAR allows students from underrepresented minority groups to have basic information about themselves distributed to the minority affairs officers of all medical schools. When these students take the MCAT, they complete a special self-identification questionnaire. Those names are placed on the Med-MAR list which is published in July and November and circulated, free of charge to the students, to all U.S. medical schools. Medical schools may then correspond with these students.

Many schools have special recruitment programs for underrepresented minorities. One prime example is Harvard Medical School (HMS), which draws 20 percent of its student body from underrepresented minorities. Harvard recruits at historically black colleges and works closely with minority student organizations. Furthermore, students who registered on the Med-MAR list receive periodic mailings. Harvard creates opportunities for underrepresented minorities to visit the school and to meet with medical students, faculty, and staff. Every spring there is a recruitment fair solely directed toward underrepresented minorities. The Office of Recruitment and Multicultural Affairs reaches out to students through mailings of brochures and posters to minority affairs officials and prehealth advisors at various colleges. If funding permits, current HMS minority students are encouraged to recruit other potential minority students during visits to their alma maters. Once accepted to HMS, minority students are invited to visit the school for a long weekend in the spring so that they will be able to meet faculty, staff, and other students.

Different medical schools have varying approaches to the admission of underrepresented minorities. While some schools have no separate minority admissions committee, they do generally attempt to have minorities interviewed by other minority members of the admissions committee. At the Stanford University School of Medicine, minority candidate applications are evaluated by two members of the admissions panel. These two members decide whether an applicant will be granted an interview. When interviews are granted, they are administered by two members of the panel. Following the interview, the application is reviewed by a minority advisory panel. Finally, the admissions committee evaluates and votes on the candidate. At the Harvard Medical School, underrepresented minority students are admitted through the regular admissions process. There is a subcommittee, consisting of students and faculty from different minority groups, that screens and evaluates these applicants. According to *Minority Student Opportunities in United States Medical Schools 1993–94,* Harvard does not have a cutoff point for GPAs and MCAT scores. In recent years, the range for science GPA has been 3.0 to 4.0, and MCAT scores have varied from eight to 15. At the Dartmouth Medical School, a subcommittee of the admissions committee reviews all minority candidates and invites strong candidates for interviews. Special attention is paid to the background of minority candidates and their involvement in the community. All minority candidates who come for interviews meet with one member of the Minority Subcommittee and with minority students as well as members of the admissions committee. The full admissions committee, which includes minorities, makes final admissions decisions.

Most schools have an academic support program available to all students — minority and non-minority. At the University of Illinois College of Medicine in Chicago, there are two minority medical school organizations which provide academic assistance to first- and second-year medical students. At the University of Miami School of Medicine there is a tutorial program for enrolled minority students who need assistance. The school also has volunteer tutors who provide one-on-one sessions and a system to identify newer students who may require such tutoring. At the University of California–San Francisco School of Medicine the UCSF Medical Scholars Program encourages minorities and women to pursue careers in academic medicine. The pursuit of excellence is championed during informal sessions in which the students present the results of their research.

Kathleen B. Lynch, Ph.D., Assistant Professor of Medical Education and Program Evaluator for the Medical Academic Advancement Program, and Moses K. Woode, Ph.D., Assistant Dean for Student Academic Support and Associate Professor of Obstetrics and Gynecology and Research Associate Professor of Chemistry, both at the University of Virginia School of Medicine, reviewed certain quantitative academic variables, specifically GPA and MCAT scores of underrepresented minority students who attended the University of Virginia School of Medicine Summer Enrichment Program. Fifty-eight of the participants applied to medical school. Of these, 49 were accepted and enrolled in 17 different medical schools. Although the authors found that the admission to medical school was not highly correlated with GPA, once admitted, all 49 of the students were retained. And they warn that quantitative variables, such as GPA and MCAT, should be used with caution when predicting the success of minority students in medical school.

Paul Jolly, Ph.D., Associate Vice President, Section for Operational Studies, AAMC, examined the acceptance rates of underrepresented minorities to medical school over the course of several years. He found that when underrepresented minorities are compared with others using similar criteria, such as the GPA and MCAT score, the minorities had substantially higher acceptance rates. As a result, Dr. Jolly concluded that schools were using affirmative action programs to attract minority applicants. Statistical data on the numbers of underrepresented minorities who apply, are accepted, and matriculate at each of the medical schools is readily available in the previously mentioned *Minority Student Opportunities in United States*

Medical Schools 1993–94. The data is presented for each school and subdivided into Black American, American Indian, Mexican American, and Mainland Puerto Rican. Then the data is subdivided again into men, women, and percent state residents. Such a presentation allows minority candidates to determine which schools attract, admit, and recruit the most minority students. It is very apparent that some schools draw far more minority candidates than others. Some have virtually no minority students. These data may help minority students and their advisors determine which schools would be more interested in minority applicants.

Although financial aid will be discussed in a future chapter, underrepresented minorities who also have limited resources should not hesitate to consider a career in medicine because of financial need. There are many financial assistance programs, scholarships, and loans. For example, the New York Medical College has a Minority Trustee Loan and scholarship award which offers $10,000 four-year scholarships and $10,000 four-year loans for entering underrepresented minority medical students. The University of Florida College of Medicine has a partial or full tuition four-year scholarship available to all entering freshman. While a medical school education was once an impossible dream for most minority students, there is no longer any reason for any interested person, who happens to be an underrepresented minority, to hesitate. Thanks to a vast array of programs designed to meet the specific needs of underrepresented minorities and the availability of financial aid, underrepresented minorities should continue to fill more of the highly coveted places at U.S. medical schools.

References — Chapter Eight

1. *Medical School Admission Requirements 1996–1997,* Association of American Medical Colleges, 1995.
2. *Minority Student Opportunities In United States Medical Schools, 1993–94,* Association of American Medical Colleges, 1993.
3. Hesser, A., Lewis, L., "Prematriculation Program Grades as Predictors of Black and Other Nontraditional Students' First-Year Academic Performances," *Academic Medicine,* 67:605–607, 1992.
4. Lynch, K.B., Woode, M.K., "The Relationship of Minority Students' MCAT Scores and Grade-Point Averages to Their Acceptance Into Medical School," *Academic Medicine,* 65:480–482, 1990.
5. Jolly, P., "Academic Achievement and Acceptance Rates of Underrepresented Minority Applicants to Medical School," *Academic Medicine,* 67:765–769, 1992.

Chapter Nine

. . . .

SPECIAL SITUATIONS

Women In Medicine

When I enrolled at Georgetown University School of Medicine in September 1968 my class had 132 students. Of these, five were women. Over the years there has been a remarkable change in the demographics of matriculating medical students and physicians.

According to the Association of American Medical Colleges (AAMC), in 1970, less than eight percent of physicians were women. Now, approximately 17 percent of physicians are women. The AAMC states in *Facts,* that in 1990, of the total applicant pool of 29,243, 40.3 percent or 11,785 were women. By 1995, when the applicant pool had risen to 45,591, 42.5 percent or 19,779 were women.

Of my two "handicaps,"

being female put many

more obstacles in my path

than being black.

Shirley Chisholm

In 1990, 6,636 or 38.7 percent of the 17,206 candidates accepted to U.S. medical schools were women. By 1995, 7,437 or 42.8 percent of the 17,357 accepted candidates were women. It is therefore not surprising that in 1990, there were 6,153 women matriculants in the first-year medical school classes. By 1995, that figure was up to 6,941. Similarly, the number of underrepresented minority women who matriculated increased from 755 in 1990 to 1,071 in 1995. Meanwhile, in 1990 there were 9,845 males matriculants. Five years later, that number was down to 9,312.

Clearly, more women are choosing to pursue a career in medicine. According to the AAMC, in the academic year 1994–95, there were several medical schools in which more than half the students were women (see Table 9-1).

Table 9-1
**Medical Schools in Which More Than Half the
Students Are Women** *(in alphabetical order)*

University of Arizona
Brown
University of California–San Francisco
University of Massachusetts
Meharry
University of Missouri–Kansas City
Morehouse
University of New Mexico
Medical College of Pennsylvania
University of Puerto Rico
University of Vermont
Wright State

Source: Medical School Admission Requirements 1996–97.

On the other hand, during the academic year 1994–95, there were schools where women represented less than 33 percent of the enrollment (see Table 9-2).

Table 9-2
**Medical Schools in Which Less Than 33 Percent
of the Enrollment Are Women** *(in alphabetical order)*

Georgetown
Louisiana State
University of Mississippi
Saint Louis
Texas Tech
Uniformed Services
University of Utah

Source: Medical School Admission Requirements 1996–1997.

At the same time, the schools, noted alphabetically in Table 9-3, reported that 50 percent or more of the entering class 1994–95 were women.

Table 9-3
Medical Schools Reporting that 50 Percent or More of the Entering Class 1994–95 Were Women *(in alphabetical order)*
University of Arizona University of California–San Francisco University of Chicago George Washington Harvard University of Hawaii Johns Hopkins University of Minnesota Northwestern University of Vermont Yale
Source: Medical School Admission Requirements 1996–1997.

During my days at Georgetown, most of the first-year class was unmarried. By our fourth year, many of us had married. Because finances were so tight, it was rare to have children. Even today, with more flexibility in curriculum and with some students spreading their medical education over more than four years, medical students rarely have children. There is generally too little money and too many years of training ahead.

Although it is frequently denied, there are still vestiges of sexual discrimination against women, especially in the areas of medicine such as general surgery, orthopedic surgery, and neurosurgery that are dominated by men. Women continue to choose residencies in internal medicine, pediatrics, and psychiatry over other fields. It may be interesting to note that I am the only male pediatrician in my department.

The Older Student

One of my pediatric practice colleagues had a first career as a teacher. It was only after she had taught for many years that she decided to become a physician. Such situations are no longer rare occurrences. More and more often people do not decide to pursue a career in medicine until several years after college. It is only then that they take the required premedical courses and enter medical school in their late 20s, 30s, or even 40s. According to an article in *Focus,* a publication of the Harvard Medical Area, the pool of applicants to the Harvard Medical School is growing older. For the class of 1999, 54 of the 166 entering students were 24 years or older. One entering student was 45 years old.

Trends Plus, a May 1994 publication of the AAMC, notes that, in terms of percentage, in 1993 there were fewer medical school applicants less than 21 years old and slightly more 28 years and older than there were in 1983. Likewise, the percentage of matriculants less than 21 years of age had fallen modestly and the percentage of matriculants age 28 or older had increased modestly between 1983 and 1993. From 1983 to 1993, the average age of matriculants had risen from 23.5 to 23.8 years. The percent of matriculants who are 28 years or older hovered slightly above ten percent for the years 1983, 1988, and 1993.

When older students decide they wish to pursue a career in medicine, they often realize that their undergraduate science preparation was woefully inadequate. For some it may be a good idea to enroll in a special postbaccalaureate premedical program. One of the oldest and most prestigious is at the Columbia University School of General Studies. The program, which has approximately 400 students, is designed for those who never studied the premedical curriculum. Literature provided by Columbia states that all applicants must have a bachelors degree with a major in an area other than the biological sciences. The minimum required grade point average (GPA) is 3.0. The Columbia program offers the premedical courses over a period of several years. Most students require two and one-half to three years to complete the coursework. While enrollment in the program does not guarantee admission to medical school, successful completion usually gives the student a solid chance at medical school acceptance.

Since 1972, Bryn Mawr College has also offered a postbaccalaureate premedical program. Materials supplied by Bryn Mawr note that the program generally requires one academic year plus one or two semesters. Over 90 percent of the those applying to medical school from this program are admitted.

There are many other schools that have formal postbaccalaureate programs. However, most colleges will allow part-time students to take the required prerequisite premedical courses. The advantage of a formal program is that it has earned a reputation and includes premedical advising and medical school counseling.

Does such postbaccalaureate education influence performance in medical school? Hoping to find an answer, Mohammadreza Hojat,

Ph.D., *et. al.*, the Director of the Jefferson Longitudinal Study at the Center for Research in Medical Education and Health Care and Assistant Professor of Psychology, Department of Psychiatry and Human Behavior, Jefferson Medical College of Thomas Jefferson University, surveyed 610 or 91 percent of the students who entered Jefferson Medical College between 1985 and 1987. According to the author, "when no adjustment is made for performance in the formal baccalaureate program, there are significant differences on some measures of performance in medical school between the students with postbaccalaureate preparation and those without such preparation, in favor of the latter group."

> *To be successful, a woman has to be much better at her job than a man.*
>
> **Golda Meir**

On the surface, these results appear logical. Those who enroll in postbaccalaureate courses probably had less undergraduate training in sciences. In addition, several years might have passed since they graduated. Nevertheless, when certain adjustments to the data were made, the differences between the groups were not significant, or, in fact, may have favored those students with some postbaccalaureate work.

The authors note that one conclusion that may be drawn from the study is that when all else is equal between traditional candidates and candidates who have received postbaccalaureate education, admissions committees should favor those who are younger with higher GPAs "but (who) also hold a graduate degree or have completed additional postbaccalaureate preparation." I disagree. In reality, postbaccalaureate students who have had various career backgrounds may contribute significantly to the mix of a medical school pool as well as the future mix of physicians.

Mary Ramsbottom-Lucier, M.D., M.P.H., an Assistant Professor in the Department of Medicine at the University of Kentucky College of Medicine, *et. al.*, compared the medical school performance of students age 28 years or older at matriculation with students 22 years or less. When compared to the younger students, the older students were found to have modestly lower GPAs. Regardless, the author maintained that the differences in GPAs "... may have been of little practical importance. ..."

The Student With Learning Disabilities

Years ago, a person with learning disabilities would not even consider applying to medical school. Today, the situation is very different. Harris Faigel, M.D., Director of University Health Services and premedical advisor at Brandeis University, surveyed 142 medical schools in the U.S. and Canada between September 1, 1990, and March 31, 1991, concerning their services and programs for students with learning disabilities. Of the 142 schools contacted, 103 returned fully completed forms. Ninety-three of the schools indicated that they accepted candidates with learning disabilities and ten did not. Interestingly, only two-thirds of the schools had support programs for students with learning disabilities and half lacked the capacity to diagnose learning disability disorders. Twenty-five of the responding schools did not even know that they could administer licensing examinations in a nonstandard manner, and 19 had no senior administrator or faculty member coordinating learning disability services. These results, the author suggests, indicate that medical schools are poorly informed about and are unprepared to help students with learning disabilities. Still, as more students with learning disabilities apply to medical schools, there will be greater pressure for medical schools to respond appropriately.

Students With Chronic Diseases or Physical Disability

Students with chronic diseases pose particularly sensitive issues for themselves as well as medical schools. When Stephan Kowalyk, M.D., was a first-year resident in internal medicine at the Cleveland Clinic, he and Harvey Hechel, M.D., an Associate Chief of Staff for Education at the Veterans Administration Medical Center, East Orange, New Jersey and Clinical Assistant Professor in the Department of Medicine, University of Medicine and Dentistry of New Jersey/New Jersey Medical School, studied the selection and performance of medical students and residents with Type I Diabetes Mellitus. According to the authors, a number of medical students and residents who have been diagnosed with Type I Diabetes Mellitus, do well in medical school. When the paper was published, many schools had no formal or informal policy regarding the acceptance of candidates with diabetes. And most schools indicated that candidates with diabetes should be treated the same as the nondiabetic candidates. Diabetes is one example of a chronic disease that is seen in some medical students. But there are others.

So having a chronic disease should not necessarily stop you from applying to medical school.

A medical student who was paralyzed from the waist down graduated from Georgetown in 1995. He sustained the disability in 1986, before matriculation at Georgetown Medical School. This new physician was able to overcome the challenges of his disability and complete a medical education.

Psychiatrically At Risk Students

Barry Willer, Ph.D., Associate Professor, Department of Psychiatry, State University of New York at Buffalo School of Medicine, *et. al.*, surveyed directors of admissions and chairs of the departments of psychiatry at U.S. and Canadian medical schools on their policies regarding the admission of psychiatrically at risk students. The authors wanted to determine if admissions committees were able to identify students with emotional problems and if psychiatrists played a role in the process. From their research, the authors concluded that the preadmission interview could be improved to identify individuals at risk for emotional problems in medical school. Chairs of the psychiatry departments were, however, less optimistic that this could be accomplished. The entire process is complicated by the fact that U.S. law "prohibits asking questions about psychiatric problems or treatments."

The issue of medical school applicants who may be psychiatrically at risk was examined further by Dr. Willer and Stuart L. Keill, M.D., Chair of the Admissions Policy Committee and Clinical Professor of Psychiatry at the State University of New York at Buffalo School of Medicine. The authors identified students at a New York medical school from 1975 to 1982 who had experienced psychiatric difficulties during their medical school career and compared them to students without psychiatric problems. Although the authors found that students who developed psychiatric problems while in medical school were similar to those who did not, ". . . there was substantially more disagreement between the interviewer ratings of students who later developed psychiatric problems than of students who did not. Presumably, at least one of the interviewers was concerned about some aspect of the student's record and/or interview. Whether these concerns were properly presented to the committee as a whole or whether the committee simply chose to ignore the concerns is not known. Schools interested in early identification of psychiatrically at risk students should look at the admissions interview as the most likely occasion for such identification."

From their research, John A. Talbott, M.D., and Robert Michels, M.D., of the Department of Psychiatry of Cornell University Medical College, have concluded that psychiatrists should become more involved in the medical school admissions process. Talbott and Michels contend that the process of admissions has three roles for psychiatrists. First, they may act as any other faculty member. Second, they may assume the role of an expert in clinical psychiatry who evaluates the ability of applicants, with known psychiatric problems, to function. Or, third, they may serve as human behavior specialists who consult with the admissions committee on certain cases.

The International Student

According to the *Medical School Admissions Requirements 1996–97*, 130 foreign students entered the first-year medical school class in 1994–95. Nevertheless, international students do encounter a number of problems when applying to U.S. medical schools. Many schools require applicants to be U.S. citizens or to hold a permanent resident visa, and state schools may have residency and citizenship requirements. In addition, since financial aid may not be available for foreign students, often they must be able to pay the entire tuition and fees. There is also the issue of fluency in English. Most successful foreign student applicants complete some undergraduate work in the U.S. If you are a foreign student, it is of particular importance to obtain information from each medical school and consult with a premedical advisor and member of the admissions committee staff.

Several medical schools accept a few foreign, non-U.S. resident students. The Harvard Medical School class of 1999 has five students who are non-U.S. residents. Foreign students may apply to Albert Einstein and the University of California–San Francisco. Some medical schools will allow foreign students to apply if they have studied in the United States. Stamford, Emory, Baylor, and Jefferson will consider foreign applicants with undergraduate preparation from a U.S. college. The amount of preparation varies from school to school, so check the requirements carefully.

Students With Disciplinary Actions

Finally, there is a small subgroup of students whose record indicates that they had disciplinary actions during their undergraduate years. Frequently, these actions are the result of a conduct violation. Should such actions prevent students from applying to medical school? The answer is a qualified no. Applicants may use the personal statement on the AMCAS form to review the violation. A minority of schools report that they use this information in admissions decisions, and there is a sense that applicants with this type of issue are accepted at half the rate of other equally qualified applicants.

To those with violations on their records, it should be of some comfort to know that schools look at applicants on a case-by-case basis. And students with violations are not automatically rejected from medical schools. If you have a violation — whether academic or disciplinary — you should be open about it on your AMCAS questionnaire, write about it in your personal statement and discuss it during the admissions interview. Never assume that such violations will, by necessity, translate into automatic rejections.

References — Chapter Nine

1. *Medical School Admission Requirements 1996–1997,* Association of American Medical Colleges, 1995.
2. *Facts,* Association of American Medical Colleges, 1995.
3. Sauber, C., "Doctor Still Has an Allure," *Focus,* September 5, 1995.
4. *Trends Plus,* Association of American Medical Colleges, 1994.
5. Hojat, M., Blacklow, R.S., Robeson, M., Veloski, J.J., Borenstein, B.D., "Postbaccalaureate Preparation and Performance in Medical School," *Academic Medicine,* 65:388–391, 1990.
6. Ramsbottom-Lucier, M., Johnson, M.M.S., Elam, C.L., "Age and Gender Differences in Students' Preadmission Qualifications and Medical School Performances," *Academic Medicine,* 70:236–239, 1995.
7. Faigel, H.C., "Services for Students With Learning Disabilities," *Academic Medicine,* 67:338–339, 1992.
8. Kowalyk, S., Hechel, H., "Selection and Performance of Medical Students and Residents With Type I Diabetes Mellitus," *Journal of Medical Education,* 61:181–183, 1986.
9. Willer, B., Keill, S., Isada, C., "Survey of U.S. and Canadian Medical Schools On Admissions and Psychiatrically At Risk Students," *Journal of Medical Education,* 59:928–936, 1984.

10. Keill, S.L., Willer, B., "Detection of Psychiatrically At Risk Applicants in the Medical School Process," *Journal of Medical Education,* 60:800–802, 1985.
11. Talbott, J., Michels, R., "The Role of Psychiatrists in the Medical School Admissions Process," *American Journal of Psychiatry,* 138:221–224, 1981.

Chapter Ten

M.D./Ph.D., Combined Baccalaureate/M.D., and Other Combination Programs

When I was in medical school, students rarely earned combination degrees. Medical students obtained M.D.'s and doctoral candidates earned their Ph.D.'s. I did not know any medical students who also planned to earn degrees in business.

As in the other areas of life, times have changed. Opportunities for students to obtain combination degrees have markedly increased. There are now many programs offering a wide range of combinations. Medical practice has become increasingly more complicated since the 1960s. There is far more diversity among the students. And diverse students bring differing interests. Students may combine a background in medicine with training in law, public policy, and business. And federal funds are now available to sponsor some M.D./Ph.D. students.

> *Two are better than one,*
>
> *for if they fall, the one will*
>
> *lift up his fellow.*
>
> **Ecclesiastes 49:10**

The most common combination program is the M.D./Ph.D. According to *Medical School Admission Requirements 1996–97,* published by the Association of American Colleges (AAMC), in 1994 to 1995 there were 113 schools that offered M.D./Ph.D. degrees. Why would a student want both medical and doctoral degrees? Generally, students who seek such a combined degree are interested in a career in academic medicine and/or research with less clinical responsibility. It would be unusual for students who expect to become clinicians, such as primary care physicians or surgeons, to devote the time or the resources to earn a doctorate.

Entering a M.D./Ph.D. program commits a student not only to the four years of medical school but also to the number of years — often four or five — necessary to complete the doctoral coursework, research, and dissertation. Thus, an M.D./Ph.D. requires about eight or nine years of post college career development. After that, the physician still has at least three years of residency. If subspecialization is desired, there are even more years of training ahead. When you start to add the number of post-high school years of education, it may come close to two decades. And that's all before beginning a career. Many people are unable to wait that long.

On the other hand, students hoping to earn an M.D./Ph.D. may have access to additional funding. Although it is beyond the scope of this book to address those funding programs, one should note that the Medical Scientist Training Program (MSTP) is available to very talented students seeking M.D./Ph.D. degrees. The MSTP provides funding, including a stipend and tuition payments, for up to six years. In the past, students incurred a payback for these funds, but since June 1993 the newly appointed trainees do not have a financial obligation. During the academic year 1994–95, the MSTP was offered at 33 U.S. medical schools, including Harvard Medical School. Harvard students may conduct research in a number of disciplines at Harvard or MIT. A Harvard M.D./Ph.D. will require a minimum of six or seven years. Frequently, it takes several years longer.

The M.D./Ph.D. degrees give research scientists the necessary training and experience to investigate human disease. Without the doctorate, physicians do not necessarily have the research background to conduct studies. It is important to note, however, that some fellowships, which are completed after residency training, include a year or more of research. Physicians who participate in such fellowships learn valuable research skills.

Bachelors/M.D. Degrees

Twenty-eight medical schools have combined baccalaureate-M.D. programs. Anthony W. Norman, Ph.D., Professor of Biochemistry at the Division of Biomedical Sciences at the University of California–Riverside, *et. al.,* notes that the first program began in 1961 at Northwestern University. Initially, the objectives of the programs were to offer an accelerated opportunity for talented high school students, reduce educational expenses, attract outstanding students to a career in medicine, and improve training in the humanities for future physicians. According to Norman, in the 1990s these programs also attempt to teach physicians to apply the liberal arts to problems in the practice of medicine, train future leaders in medicine, graduate physicians who understand the intricacies of technology applied to medicine, and prepare physicians for community medicine.

Though the programs vary in length from six to eight years, they all require four years of medical training. A small number have only two years of undergraduate coursework. Students in those programs complete their undergraduate and medical school training in six years. Assuming they continue to do good work, students who decide to enter such programs from high school are assured entrance into medical school. In addition, time and tuition fees may be saved. On the other hand, shortening the undergraduate years — a time to receive a well-rounded classical education — may be a decided disadvantage, and some high school students may feel that they are too young to commit to a specific medical school.

Some schools, such as New York University School of Medicine, only accept a handful of high school students for their program. Other schools, such as the Northeastern Ohio University College of Medicine, primarily offer a combined B.S.–M.D. curriculum to honors high school graduates.

According to Stanley W. Olson, M.D., a Consultant in Medical Education and Distinguished Service Member of the AAMC, the academic performance of combined degree students is as good as or better than those following the traditional undergraduate/medical school pathway. "Early bloomers," high schoolers with definite career goals who are committed to the life pursuit of medicine, may be particularly attracted to such programs.

For high school students who rank high in their class and have strong college entrance examination SAT scores, Howard University has a program leading to a bachelor's degree and a M.D. degree from the College of Medicine at Howard University. During the first two years, students focus on undergraduate work. The remaining four years are devoted to medical studies. Twenty-five applicants applied to the 1994–95 entering class; ten entered.

Boston University has a similar program. Like Howard, students are selected in the senior year of high school. Though the Boston University program averages seven years in length, there are six- and eight-year options. In the class beginning 1994–95, there were 868 applicants. Twenty-three entered.

Other Combination Degrees

While the M.D./Ph.D. is by far the most common combination degree, there are other intriguing combinations. For those interested in oral and maxillofacial surgery, the University of California–San Francisco, School of Medicine, offers a D.D.S./M.D. Yale University combines a medical degree with a master's in divinity (M.D./M.Div.).

Those concerned with the increasingly complex management of health care systems may wish to consider one of the schools that combine a M.D. with a management or business degree. For example, Northwestern University offers the M.D.– M.M. (Master of Management), and the University of Pennsylvania has the M.D.–M.B.A. (Master of Business Administration). These programs provide a background in health care administration and may lead to a career as director of a medical organization.

Duke University offers a program that combines the M.D. with a master's in public policy. Such a degree is preparation for work in the public arena. A small number of schools combine the M.D. degree with the J.D. or law degree. An attorney with a medical degree could have a decided advantage in certain aspects of trial law involving complex medical issues.

Harvard and several other schools have programs that combine the M.D. degree with the M.P.H. or master's in public health. Hence, Harvard Medical School students who wish to take a break from their medical school studies may earn a Harvard M.P.H. in nine months.

Such programs give students solid backgrounds in statistics and epidemiology. Johns Hopkins University has an M.D.–Doctor of Public Health program that provides an outstanding background for an academic position in public health.

Finally, a number of schools consolidate medical studies with a master's of science degree. At the University of Maryland students may combine their M.D. degree with an M.S. in epidemiology.

Most medical schools have special programs that do not necessarily lead to degrees. One uniquely creative example is the Harvard–MIT Program in Health Sciences and Technology — a program designed to educate physician/scientists. Although some of the students who participate in this program earn an M.D./Ph.D., most do not earn combination degrees. The coursework unites the resources of Harvard and MIT with students who have strong backgrounds in quantitative and biological sciences. According to Luann Wilkerson, Ed.D., former Director of Faculty Development,

Harvard Medical School, and Walter H. Abelmann, M.D., Professor of Medicine, emeritus, Harvard Medical School, the first class of 25 medical students were admitted to the Harvard–MIT Program in Health Sciences and Technology in 1971. Between 1975 and 1985, 234 students graduated. Two hundred and eleven or 90 percent responded to a survey administered by Wilkerson and Abelmann. According to the authors, of the 211 students, 63 or 30 percent, earned both M.D. and Ph.D. degrees. The graduates of the program were more likely to be in academic rather than clinical practice. Ninety-four held full-time faculty positions at 50 medical schools. One hundred and fifty-four, or 73 percent, devoted an average of 51 percent of their time to research. Most of the program's graduates entered medicine as a career path; only 13 of the 211 students did not.

It is quite obvious that there are a number of different career paths available to those who seek combination degrees. Without a doubt, holders of these degrees have expanded marketability and the flexibility to enter several career paths. The opportunities seem endless. But that is all part of the enticement and excitement in medicine today.

References — Chapter Ten

1. *Medical School Admission Requirements 1996–1997,* Association of American Medical Colleges, 1995.
2. *1994–95 Curriculum Directory,* Association of American Medical Colleges, 1994.
3. *Minority Student Opportunities in United States Medical Schools 1993–94,* Association of American Medical Colleges, 1993.
4. Norman, A.W., Calkins, E.V., "Curriculum Variations in Combined Baccalaureate-M.D. Programs," *Academic Medicine,* 67:785–791, 1992.
5. Olson, S.W., "Combined-degree Programs: A Valuable Alternative for Motivated Students Who Choose Medicine Early," *Academic Medicine,* 67:783–784, 1992.
6. Wilkerson, L., Abelmann, W.H., "Producing Physician-Scientists: A Survey of Graduates From Harvard-MIT Program in Health Sciences and Technology," *Academic Medicine,* 68:214–218, 1993.

Chapter 11
. . . .

MEDICAL SCHOOL SELECTION

Congratulations! You have been accepted to medical school. Consider yourself very fortunate.

If you have been admitted to only one school, you really have no choice. That is the medical school you will attend.

On the other hand, if you have received more than one offer, you must now make a very important decision. It is perhaps one of the most momentous decisions of your life and one that will play a pivotal role in your future growth as a physician.

The finely detailed rules governing the acceptance procedures — the so called "traffic rules" — are published yearly by the Association of American Medical Colleges (AAMC) in "Medical School Admissions Requirements." These recommend that candidates hold no more than one medical school acceptance. Thus, a medical school applicant who receives acceptances from two or more schools should accept the "pre-

"Yes," I answered you
. . . .
last night, "no," this
. . . .
morning, sir, I say colors
. . . .
seen by candlelight will
. . . .
not look the same by day.

Elizabeth Barrett Browning

ferred" school as soon as possible and notify the other school(s) of this decision. These rules, as well as the general AAMC guidelines and materials from the medical schools to which you have been accepted, should all be carefully reviewed.

How should you decide which medical school to attend? Sometimes, the process is rather easy. You are accepted by your first choice school. Often, however, that is not the case. So how do you make a decision?

For most students, the crucial guiding factor is reputation. But how does one determine the reputation of a particular school? Such distinctions are not always clear cut. Consult your premedical advisor. He or she may have had experience with former advisees who have decided to attend the schools you are considering. Contact physicians who graduated from the schools or who may know about the reputations of various schools. That is, however, only the beginning. Undoubtedly, you are aware that there are published assessments of medical schools. One of the most famous is the *U.S. News & World Report* annual review of medical and other graduate schools. The *U.S. News & World Report* data is developed, in part, by surveying senior medical school officials throughout the country. In establishing the rank order of research-oriented medical schools, this survey looked at the following areas:

1. Reputation ranked by academics
2. Reputation ranked by intern/residency directors
3. Student selectivity index
4. Faculty resource rank
5. Research activity rank
6. Average '94 MCAT score
7. '94 Acceptance rate
8. '94 Total NIH research
9. Faculty student ratio
10. '94 Out-of-state tuition

In the *U.S. News & World Report* the schools are divided into the 25 highest ranked research-oriented medical schools and the 14 highest ranked primary care-oriented medical schools. Further, in the magazine's most recent report, dated March 20, 1995, it also ranked schools by specialty. For example, the magazine listed the five best schools in the following eight categories: AIDS Research, Drug and Alcohol Abuse, Family Medicine, Geriatric Care, Internal Medicine, Pediatrics, Rural Medicine, and Women's Health.

While these ratings may help you make a decision, do not use them as the primary criteria for selecting a medical school. A careful review of the surveys shows that some are based on subjective opinions of academics or intern/residency directors. Also, there are schools in urban locations that have far more faculty involvement or better faculty/student ratios. And although MCAT scores are quoted for the various top-ranked schools, as you have already read in this book, there are other factors that schools may take into account when deciding the composition of a class. It would be the rare school that accepted a student solely on the basis of a high MCAT score.

Although the report divides medical schools between those that are research-oriented — and heavily subsidized by the National Institutes of Health — and those that focus on primary care, it should not be forgotten that a good clinical background may be acquired at a research-oriented medical school, and a solid academic education may be obtained from a school with a high rating in primary care. Moreover, there are many medical schools not ranked in either research-oriented or primary care categories that offer a fine medical education. It is significant to note that some of the differences in ranks were numerically quite small. Most of the nation's medical schools should provide a thorough medical education. Nonetheless, according to the *U.S. News & World Report,* the breakdown of the research-oriented medical schools were as indicated in Table 11-1.

The *U.S. News & World Report* used the following factors to rank

---

Table 11-1
Top-Ranked Research-Oriented Medical Schools

1. Harvard
2. Johns Hopkins
3. Yale
4. Duke
5. Washington University
6. University of California–San Francisco
7. University of Pennsylvania
8. Columbia
9. Cornell
10. University of Michigan–Ann Arbor
11. University of Washington
12. Stanford
13. University of California–Los Angeles
14. University of California–San Diego
15. Vanderbilt
16. Baylor
17. University of Pittsburgh
18. University of Chicago
19. University of Texas SW Medical Center–Dallas
20. Yeshiva/Albert Einstein College of Medicine
21. Case Western Reserve
22. Mayo
23. Emory
24. University of Alabama–Birmingham
25. New York University

Source: U.S. News & World Report.

the primary care-oriented medical schools:
1. Reputation ranked by academics
2. Reputation ranked by intern/residency directors
3. Student selectivity rank
4. Faculty resource rank
5. Primary care rank
6. Percent of graduates in primary care
7. Average '94 MCAT score
8. '94 Acceptance rate
9. Faculty/student ratio
10. '94 Out-of-state tuition

Again, several of these criteria were subjective, particularly the reputation ranks. Even so, they were ranked as noted in Table 11-2.

Another way to assess the reputations of various medical schools is to request lists of the internship placements for their graduates. You may then refer to the hospital rankings compiled by *U.S. News & World Report* to determine if the medical school is placing its graduates in the top hospitals. You may also consult with other physicians for their opinions.

Remember, these rankings are often based on subjective or semi-

---

Table 11-2
Top-Ranked Primary Care Medical Schools

1. University of Washington
2. University of California–Davis
3. Michigan State
3. University of Kentucky (there was a tie here)
5. University of Iowa
6. University of Massachusetts–Worcester
7. University of New Mexico
8. University of Texas Health Science Center–San Antonio
9. East Carolina
10. University of Missouri–Columbia
11. University of Minnesota–Duluth
12. Oregon
13. University of Colorado
14. University of California–San Francisco
15. Thomas Jefferson — Jefferson Medical

Source: U.S. News & World Report.

subjective factors. For example, examine a copy of *U.S. News & World Report,* July 12, 1993. To establish the ranking of the hospitals in pediatrics, the magazine used five criteria — the reputational score (based on the number of surveyed doctors who named the hospital), the ratio of board certified pediatricians to number of hospital beds, the technology score (an index from 1 to 19), the ratio of registered nurses to number of beds, and whether the hospital is a member of the Council of Teaching Hospitals (COTH). From these, the magazine determined that the facilities indicated in Table 11-3 were the five top-ranked hospitals in pediatrics.

Table 11-3
Top-Ranked Pediatric Centers

1. Children's Hospital, Boston
2. Children's Hospital of Philadelphia
3. Johns Hopkins Hospital
4. Children's Hospital of Los Angeles
5. Children's Hospital of Pittsburgh

Source: U.S. News & World Report.

Similarly, in 1994, *U.S. News & World Report* named the 12 best hospitals in the country. The top five hospitals are cited in Table 11-4.

Again, please use these rankings as only one piece of information. Certainly do not consider them an absolute guide to the quality of hospitals.

Many students view location — the region of the country and whether the medical school is located in an urban, suburban, or

---

Table 11-4
Top-Ranked Hospitals

1. Johns Hopkins Hospital
2. Mayo Clinic
3. UCLA Medical Center
4. Massachusetts General Hospital
5. Duke University Medical Center

Source: U.S. News & World Report.

rural setting — as an important consideration when selecting a medical school. The number of hospital beds is also worthy of note. If few beds are available to medical schools, then you will have less opportunity to interact with hospitalized patients. On the other hand, if larger numbers of beds are open to medical students, then your chances for interaction with patients will be enhanced. As you continue your investigation, try to learn more about the facilities used by the medical school. How many hospitals are affiliated with the medical school? In which of these hospitals do the medical students rotate? Do the rotations permit a certain degree of flexibility? In other words, under certain circumstances, are you able to create your own rotation?

For the vast majority of medical students, the cost of medical school is a critical factor. Some students enter medical school already in debt from their undergraduate education. Now they are faced with four more years of tuition and living expenses. Since medical school is often followed by years of low paid training, generally it is some time before young physicians are able to make meaningful repayments on loans. If you attend a private medical school, you may easily incur tens of thousands of dollars — even well over a hundred thousand dollars — in loans. Some physicians who have amassed such heavy debt may feel compelled to enter higher paying specialties while physicians who attend less expensive medical schools may have more freedom to enter lower paying areas of medicine. Usually, the state medical schools cost less than the private medical schools. And, in fact, some state schools have programs in which the tuition is waived or partially waived when a student commits to practicing certain specialties in the state.

Frequently, the situation is not that simple. Sometimes, private schools offer a higher financial aid package than a public school. Ironically, it may be less expensive to attend a private school with an excellent financial aid package than a state school with less generous resources. Do not forget to add the cost of transportation to and from school as well as books, instruments, supplies, and the necessities of life. The whole issue of cost and financial aid will be discussed in greater detail in the next chapter.

Let's assume you have narrowed your selection to two choices, and you still are unable to make a decision. Perhaps it is time to pay more attention to programming. Contact the admissions offices and ask them for the most recent material on programs available at the schools. There could be a special course or offering that helps you make a decision. You should also consult the *Curriculum Directory,* published by the AAMC, which details and categorizes the programming of each medical school. Thus, the *Curriculum Directory* lists the required courses such as lectures, conferences, and small group laboratories, and the numbers of hours that students are expected to spend in each of these. It further notes information on the required clerkships completed during the third and fourth years. Of particular interest are data on the grading system of each school and listings of which schools require students to pass the United States Medical Licensing Exam (USMLE) Step I and Step II.

You could also be attracted to a particular school because it has an innovative curriculum. Gordon T. Moore, M.D., M.P.H., Director of Teaching Programs at Harvard Community Health Plan and Associate Professor in the Department of Ambulatory Care and Prevention at Harvard Medical School, *et. al.,* described the New Pathway (NP) curriculum at Harvard Medical School (HMS). The NP places a select group of preclinical students into a program with three main objectives. First, it provides students with an adequate background in biomedicine. Second, it teaches students the skills needed to become humanistic physicians who deliver patient care by integrating biological principles with social and behavioral concepts. And, third, it offers instruction in self-directed learning. Some of the methods used to reach these goals include problem-based learning, intense small-group interactions, and participation in a longitudinal patient-doctor relationship that integrates clinical skill development with ethics, preventive medicine, and the social and behavioral sciences.

According to Dr. Moore, when compared to students in the traditional curriculum, the NP students learn differently, acquire a unique body of knowledge, skills, and attitudes, and have a more satisfying and challenging preclinical experience. NP students had no loss of biomedical competence.

There is still another area where you may turn for help. Many premedical offices ask former students to complete questionnaires on the medical schools they attend. Generally, these are compiled in some organized format in the office and may give valuable, subjective opinions of the different schools. To learn even more, you may even wish to telephone or visit one or two of the students. Thanks to my years of premedical advising at MIT, I have a host of former students who are now attending medical schools. I asked several of them to reply to a survey form. Consider them a helpful adjunct to your decision-making process.

The following questions were sent to all the students:

1. What are the school's best qualities? Include teaching, loca-

tion, students, competition, academic quality, patients, costs, and whatever else you would like to say.

2. What are some bad qualities that come to mind?

3. If you had a chance, would you attend the same school and why?

4. Feel free to use the remaining room on this side and the back for any other comments about the school

HARVARD MEDICAL SCHOOL

1 • Excellent faculty (both preclinical and clinical), many truly dedicated to teaching.
• Superb facilities — accessible to students 24 hours a day (computers, histo lab, anatomy lab, etc.).
• Diverse, interesting student body.
• Great location (Boston — fun, pretty safe place to be).
• PASS/FAIL for years 1 and 2 (makes for less competition among classmates).

2 • Tutorial-based New Pathway is not for everyone Courses in years three and four are tough to get where and when you want them.
• HMS is an expensive place to go, and Boston is an expensive place to live!
• In third and fourth years, probably not enough exposure to community-based outpatient medicine

3   Definitely. I think the first two years were a lot less painful at HMS than at more traditional medical schools, and the third and fourth years with rotations at places like Brigham and Women's Hospital, Mass. General Hospital, Beth Israel, and Children's Hospital are ***great***. I think there are few med schools where students interact with (and learn from) some of the best clinicians and scientists in the U.S. and have a pretty good time doing so.

JOHNS HOPKINS

1 • Hopkins' good reputation opens opportunities for research and academic careers for its graduates.
• First year is not as demanding as in other schools at Hopkins, classes are 8:00 a.m.–1 p.m. during the first year.

• Hopkins provides excellent access to patients with diverse problems.

2 • Those who are more clinically oriented may find Hopkins too research focused.
• The school is located in a part of the city where crime is very high.

3 Absolutely yes. The benefits of attending a school of such a reputation outweighs the weakness of the program.

UNIVERSITY OF CALIFORNIA, SAN FRANCISCO

1 • Teaching — excellent, enthusiastic, caring professors who will spend time with you if you really need extra help.
• Teachers — very open and receptive and responsive to criticism for changes.
• Cost — very low.
• Location — San Francisco, California, exciting, urban, great variety of patients.
• Students — diversity.
• Different schools and majors.
• You are competitive with yourself not with others.
• You want to do well, students work together.
• Pass/Fail first year.
• Wednesdays are off so you can do community service or research.

2 • Sometimes the Administration's paternalistic attitude (e.g., Honors is necessary in the second year even if you, the students, don't think so).
• Housing expensive.
• Nowhere to park.
• No lockers.

3 Yes. Location. Students (great diversity — different ages, races, socioeconomic status — very intelligent), teaching great.

UNIVERSITY OF ROCHESTER

1 The school's best quality is that from day one we are taught that as doctors we will be treating people, not just their illnesses. This is emphasized through patient contact from the first week of classes, specific classes and discussion on the doctor-patient relationship, and classes in human development and psychology. Even throughout the core clinical/ science courses we are constantly reminded that the reason we're here is to help people — not just to be fascinated by their pathology. In keeping with this focus, first-year students are required to take medical humanities classes ranging from literature and philosophy to ethics and law. While some may be thrilled to never take a humanities course again after college, I've really enjoyed these classes, the discussion they've encouraged amongst classmates and have found them a welcome change from the rest of the science curriculum. Most of the teachers here are really great! Dr. XXX, the first instructor to be encountered in Anatomy is terrific and I think the best lecturer I've ever had. Most of the faculty really is dedicated to teaching, welcome feedback, and are very approachable — the histology and neuroscience professors have been known to come to our parties and join students going out for beers! At MIT I skipped many a lecture — usually because it wasn't really beneficial. Here, even though classes start at 8 a.m. I hardly ever miss a lecture — they really are taught well and are worth going to. I guess a lot of the information is the same wherever it's being taught but I can honestly say I know I'm being taught well here.

The class is also really great. There are 99 in the class — 40 women, 59 men. I didn't expect as much diversity as there is — no, its not quite like MIT. But there really is a broad representation of races, backgrounds, and academic experiences. The class is also very united — even after seeing each other every day during the week we often get together on the weekend to go out and yes, study. There have been many parties, ski trips, dinners — its hard to be antisocial with this group. While school is everyone's priority, we seem to do a pretty good job of having some fun. I feel really lucky to know I'll be working with this group of people for the next few years and maybe even the rest of my life. Of course, there is some competitiveness. But I think that's to be expected when you put 100 ambitious people together. The administration fosters a very relaxed learning environment. For me, my own desire to do well has been what's pushed me — not anyone else's grades or competition.

About Rochester, I really like it! If you enjoy the outdoors this place is great. There's a lot of country parks to sled, hike, and cross-country ski. The beautiful Finger Lakes are an hour away and if you want a big city, Toronto is three hours away. No, Rochester is not a hip-happening cultural mecca but you can easily grow to like it.

2   The worst quality for many people is Rochester as a city. There's not a lot of sun, there is a lot of snow, you *need* a car to get around, 8.5 percent sales tax on everything, no more Newbury St. or Charles River, and not really too exciting if you're into the big-city environment. But, as I said, if you like the outdoors, this place is beautiful and can be a lot of fun!

3   Honestly, the school is pretty great and I'm really happy to be here. I would most definitely come to the U of R all over again. It's not for everyone though. Some people think they focus too much on the "biopsychosocial" aspect of medicine (yeah, that's a big buzz word around here — it means what it says.) But I personally feel that with all the changes occurring in medicine today, as doctors in training, we have to be aware of the world around us and not just of medicine as a science.

YALE

1   Yale is on a Pass/Fail (no high pass) system. This allows us to study and learn at our own pace. Competition between students is almost nonexistent. The costs are comparable to most other private institutions. The faculty is skilled in relating concepts/information. They are dedicated and eager. There is also a clinical tutor assigned to a group of four students. This group meets weekly to "round" on specific patients. Much of the material during the first two years is clinically-oriented as well as basic sciences-centered. There are plenty of research opportunities and a thesis program.

2   Pass/Fail system could allow the student to fall behind and not study intensely. The class curriculum/schedule can be confusing in that the academic planning office frequently reschedules and tries to combine classes toward an "integrated" curriculum. The school is located in New Haven, CT — bad neighborhood, almost no social life.

3   Yes. Yale graduates place very well for residency. The P/F system allowed me to be selective about what I felt was necessary to learn and retain. My main complaint — *the location.*

NORTHWESTERN

1   Downtown location, lake, new curriculum's goals (fewer lecture hours), emphasis on clinical aspects and patient care, closeness to my home, problem-based learning

2   Class is too large (170 students), some problems with new curriculum (this is the second year of it), cliques from those in the seven-year Honors program at Northwestern (which make it difficult only in the very beginning).

3   Yes, because the new curriculum gives me time to do other things besides sit in class. However, I wonder if I am learning enough.

4   The new curriculum, although good in its intentions, expects too much of students. We are required to photocopy lecture notes at the library after lecture instead of having them given to us. This is to promote "self-directed" learning.

TUFTS

1   For the most part, teaching at Tufts is quite good especially in the important clinical subjects. Students are informed of the latest research results and clinical investigations. Location-wise Tufts students actually have the benefits of seeing illnesses among the Asian immigrants which don't occur much in the U.S. Although the students are quite private with their grades and evaluations, they are quite willing to help one another with their studies. I find the curriculum is well planned and provides more than adequate preparation for the board exams and third-year clinical rotations, provided one can maintain the learned material.

2 One particular weakness about Tufts is its cost/tuition which is overwhelming. However, the school is very supportive about helping students to attain the best types of loans.

3 Yes, I would attend the same school because despite the high loan debt at the end of fours years, Tufts has provided me with an education that hopefully will prepare me well to become a competent clinician.

UNIVERSITY OF SOUTHERN CALIFORNIA

1 Gross Anatomy is very well taught in year one! The pathology department also excels in teaching throughout year two. There is a friendly atmosphere around the relationships with other students; everyone is intense about academics, but competition is not really evident. ICM (Intro to Clinical Medicine) in years one and two are exceptional for giving hands-on interaction with patients and preparing diagnostic skills for rotations.

2 Campus location (high crime area), tuition costs, library isn't open 24 hours. Not enough time to study for boards (three weeks at end of year two).

3 Yes. I was definitely looking for a school that was clinically-oriented, and USC fits that bill. California is great, and L.A. County is a fantastic teaching hospital. And L.A. is a great city to explore outside of medical school.

NEW YORK UNIVERSITY

1

New York University has excellent teaching in anatomy, neuroscience medicine, histology, and pathology. The third- and fourth-year rotations are also taught very well by the attending staff. Location is a plus since it is in Manhattan and easily accessible to a variety of entertainment. Classes are structured to be very noncompetitive. Only P/F. No honors or high pass grades for first and second years. Wide variety of patients in three teaching hospitals. However, tuition is very high, $25,000, and housing is also expensive. My class had 100 percent passing for the National Boards Part I.

2 Expensive tuition and board. Patients at Bellevue provide good academic experience, but are not often very pleasant people. Brutal.

GEORGE WASHINGTON

1 • Noncompetitive.
• Washington D.C. — lots of recreational opportunities, research, hospitals.
• Interaction with faculty excellent.
• Primary care apprenticeships expose students to clinical medicine beginning the first year.

2 Cost. I don't think you get your moneys worth.

3 No. I think I would have gone to my state school.

HARVARD MEDICAL SCHOOL (M.D./Ph.D. PROGRAM)

1 The resources at Harvard Medical School, in particular with respect to the M.D./Ph.D. program, are quite impressive. Clinically, students are able to choose elective subjects from several hospitals encompassing a very broad range of medical fields; the medical school maintains an active exchange program which generally makes it possible to find a rotation if it is not available here. From a research point of view, opportunities abound to do molecular biology as well as clinically-relevant basic research as a medical student. Ph.D. students are able to work in laboratories at the Harvard campus in Cambridge as well as MIT.

The New Pathway program, which has a reduced number of hours of instruction compared to other programs, gives students greater flexibility in focusing on those areas of medical education they deem most personally important and relevant. Many students make use of this time by going into the standard areas of instruction in greater depth, or by doing research, community medicine, outreach, etc. Thus, this program is not well suited to students who do not have a self-directed and self-motivated style of learning.

Harvard medical students come from a broad range of background and interests. In general, they are talented and dynamic, which facilitates students teaching each other — a common event in the New Pathway. In general, overall teaching and course organization, both basic science and clinical, ranges from good to excellent.

2   The sheer size of Harvard is overwhelming at times, and navigating the administrative seas can be challenging. The "flexibility" of the program is viewed by some as a lack of direction, and students may feel lost or fear that they are studying the wrong topics. It is, in fact, possible to come away from a course without having mastered all the major topics because there is a scarcity of direct supervision and no grades (first two years are Pass/Fail and almost everyone passes). The perspective of the basic science faculty tends to be very academic and very cutting edge. Thus, some students complain that they are taught detailed molecular topics at the expense of more basic practical information. There exists here, as at all medical schools, the tendency for faculty to discuss their own personal research topics without giving due attention to the broader areas of their fields. However, the limited number of class hours in the first two years helps to ensure that a higher percentage of faculty give well-prepared lectures that cover wide areas.

The New Pathway program involves an emphasis on case-based education in small groups, which can lead to an excessive amount of time being spent discussing simple group dynamics. The students at Harvard, being the talented group that they are, do sometimes come with baggage that can make these small group discussions difficult. Finally, cost is a major issue. M.D./Ph.D. students do not pay tuition and receive a small stipend, but admission to this program (as well as the medical school at large) is highly competitive.

3   In my next life: If I had it to do over again, as someone interested in a career in academic medicine and bench research, I would definitely still choose Harvard. The opportunities to do research, even during the first two years, and the flexibility to choose among so many options were and still are the most important factors in my decision.

UNIVERSITY OF CALIFORNIA–
SAN FRANCISCO (M.D./Ph.D. PROGRAM)

1
- Teaching — is outstanding. A great deal of effort is put in by the faculty. Recently, an instructor stayed with us in anatomy lab till two in the morning.
- Location — San Francisco is a great city with nice weather.
- Students — I feel close with everyone in my class. I'm very impressed by their compassion, intelligence, and friendliness.
- Competition — It isn't a huge problem, but every class tends to be different. Among my friends there is a great deal of helping and group studying.
- Academic quality — UCSF has a good academic reputation.
- Patients — We see patients in the first year. UCSF is lucky to have affiliations with top hospitals like San Francisco General.
- Costs — Compared to MIT, it's a bargain — even for out-of-state. But in the future, it looks as though costs will rise due to California's strapped budget.

2   None really come to mind.

3   Yes. I couldn't be happier for the reasons above.

YALE MEDICAL SCHOOL

1   Around here "The Yale System" is a catch phrase that can mean almost anything and is used to emphasize many points. It means we are not ranked, not graded, we are not even reduced to a number because the numbers we are assigned (and by which we take our exams) are not revealed to the administration. This atmosphere lends itself to noncompetitive interaction among students and avoids "forced attendances" in classes and small sections. If you don't like something, or you have something better to do, you can leave class. The Yale System does not revolve around exams or deadlines. It creates an environment that will (hopefully) last for the rest of a physician's career, that is, an environment of stable and sustained learning in addition to the pursuit of other interests and goals.

Yale encourages research which is great because they fund

your first summer of research. If you can find an advisor/ sponsor, they will fund almost anything — wet lab stuff, clinical, literature (somewhat medically related), whatever. It's a great option because many students do outstanding research and manage to publish while in medical school.

The patient population here is mostly inner city and under-privileged which is an advantage for the medical student because you'll get to see many varied diseases that have progressed to a more advanced stage than the same disease in an affluent setting.

As far as I remember, Yale's tuition and fees were at the low end of the private medical school spectrum. Also keep in mind that for the first year summer they fund $2,200 to do research many students would probably volunteer to do.

2   New Haven is not a great place to live. There is one movie theatre in town, and about a dozen restaurants that are good and make a nice night out. Yale has every art and music and drama outlet you can think of but I still miss an active living like Boston or, my hometown, New York City.

3   I would *only* attend Yale, having been a happy and satisfied student here I really couldn't imagine having endless hours of classes. (Yale has the fewest class hours of any medical school), plus trying to study for exams (Yale's exams are anonymous until the second term of the second year at which point they are essentially optional). And contrary to what you many think could happen, there really aren't any abuses of the system and everyone is motivated and above all well balanced.

UNIVERSITY OF SOUTHERN CALIFORNIA

1   The clinical experience is fabulous. During the first two years every student goes to the hospital once a week as part of a course (Introduction to Clinical Medicine I and II). The history and physical exams are practiced on a regular basis and is given much focus. Students can also go to the hospital at their own leisure and practice. All the physicians are very helpful in teaching. Third- and fourth-year students have an extensive hands-on experience. Interns that went to USC Medical School are clearly more experienced than many from other schools.

2 • There is too much class time — often 8 a.m. to 5 p.m. every day.
  • There is not enough time to study for boards (two to three weeks).

3 Yes. I love the clinical experience; the students are great. The weather is fabulous and LA is lots of fun.

DUKE UNIVERSITY

1 • Handouts are given for almost all lectures. Great services — videotapes, lectures, and help available by the professors.
  • Diverse class. Some were lawyers, many took a year off or worked for several years. Few received Ph.D.'s.
  • Location. Durham, North Carolina. Not much to do if you do not have a car. Nearby cities (Chapel Hill) are where people go out at night at times.
  • More slow-paced than cities like NYC or Boston.

2 • Classes are too crammed (similar to crash courses).
  • Fast-paced, not difficult material to learn, but a little too much material to try to memorize and have firm grasp of.

3 Great opportunity to do research (third year); however, I may choose a different school closer to home and where pace of life is a little faster.

References — Chapter Eleven

1. *Medical School Admission Requirements 1996–1997,* Association of American Medical Colleges, 1995.
2. "Medical Schools," *U.S. News & World Report,* March 20, 1995.
3. "America's Best Hospitals," *U.S. News & World Report,* July 12, 1993.
4. *U.S. News & World Report,* July 10, 1993.
5. *Curriculum Directory 1994–1995,* Association of American Medical Colleges, 1994.
6. Moore, G.T., Block, S.O., Style, C.B., Mitchell, R., "The Influence of the New Pathway Curriculum on Harvard Medical Students," *Academic Medicine,* 69:983–989, 1994.

Chapter Twelve
. . . .

FINANCING A MEDICAL SCHOOL EDUCATION

In 1968, when I graduated from college, I was debt free. Thanks to a host of different jobs, I had paid for my entire undergraduate education at a state university.

Unfortunately, my financial situation was far from secure. In a few months I was scheduled to begin medical school, and my savings account had less than $500. I had been able to save only a fraction of what I would need. Nevertheless, even more jobs and a variety of funding sources enabled me to complete medical school in four years. Many of these financial resources, which proved invaluable at the time, are still available.

It has always been my belief that the lack of financial backing should never be a reason not to apply to medical school. In fact, if the physicians of the future are to represent all segments of society, including the economically disadvantaged, there must be mechanisms in place to welcome all qualified candidates without regard for the ability to pay.

> *The only thing more*
> . . . .
> *expensive than*
> . . . .
> *education is ignorance.*
>
> **Benjamin Franklin**

In this chapter, I hope to present an overview of some of the programs available to medical students and to offer a preliminary introduction to financial assistance. It would, however, be to your advantage to look beyond what I say and to conduct more research of your own. When my wife and I were dating, we would often spend hours in the library researching scholarship and loan opportunities. While that did not make for very exciting dates, it enabled me to locate some of the less well-known sources. Remember, when it comes to financing your medical education, think creatively.

Unless you are one of the small number of medical students whose family is willing and able to pay for your entire education, costs will be part of your medical school selection decision. There is a significant variation in costs between private and public medical schools. And some schools are more heavily endowed with scholarship funds than others. As a future medical student, you should be researching this information.

It is important to note that borrowing to pay for your education impacts your future earnings. In a sense, by borrowing you are gambling that your medical education and future training and job positions will generate sufficient income to cover the debt and interest.

Today, the tuition at the most expensive medical schools is around $31,000 per year. The average (mean) tuition for the private schools is about $23,000. To this figure you must add the cost of living, room and board, supplies and other materials, and perhaps the use of a car. Together they may total another $12,000. Thus, the average yearly cost to attend a private medical school ranges from $34,000 to more than $40,000. Students attending a private medical school who are already in debt from their undergraduate years could easily end up owing $200,000 or more. According to *Focus,* a publication of the Harvard Medical School Office of Public Affairs, of the 152 graduates in the Harvard Medical School Class of 1995, 109 students had outstanding loans. The average medical school debt for these new physicians was $66,231. Faced with such an astounding debt, some students may be unwilling to consider entering some of the lower paid areas of medicine, such as primary care or academic medicine. As I said in Chapter 11 (Medical School Selection), it is possible that your choice of medical school, specialization, or career could be influenced by unpaid loans.

So what are some of the financial aid programs available to medical students and how may they be accessed? The process of applying for financial aid begins with the **Free Application for Federal Student Aid (FAFSA)**. This application, designed by the U.S. Department of Education Student Financial Assistance Program, has several sections. It will request general demographic information about you, your educational background and future plans, your sources of income, and past loans. Complete it fully and send it by mail to the processing center as soon as possible after January 1.

In general, the FAFSA application determines eligibility for several different federal programs including the **Pell Grants, Stafford Loans, Supplemental Educational Opportunity Grants (SEOG),** and **Federal Work-Study**. Among other requirements, students must be U.S. citizens or eligible noncitizens.

All medical schools participate in the **Federal Stafford Loan**

Program. This federally subsidized program is available to medical students with financial need. Currently, the loans are limited to $8,500 per academic year. The total amount of Stafford indebtedness, which may include debt incurred during your undergraduate years, may not exceed $138,500. Depending on financial need, the rates may or may not be subsidized. The interest rate for both types of loans has been capped at 8.25 percent. At present, students are required to begin repayment six months after medical school graduation.

The Federal Perkins Loan Program is available to medical students who are U.S. citizens or eligible noncitizens. Perkins loans are low-interest loans awarded by the medical school's financial aid office. Each medical school has a certain amount allocated for this program. Most recently, the interest rate was 5 percent. Unless deferred, payments begin six months after graduation. Medical students may receive up to $30,000 of Perkins loans, including money borrowed during the undergraduate years. In medical school, a maximum of $5,000 in Perkins loans may be borrowed each year.

The Health Profession Student Loan Program (HPSL), also sponsored by the federal government, has limited resources and is available only to the most needy. The financial aid offices of the medical schools determine the amounts of the loans. Each year, students may borrow the cost of tuition plus $2,500. At present, the rate of interest is 5 percent. The principal and interest may be deferred during medical training and military service.

Unlike the previously noted programs, the **Health Education Assistance Loan Program (HEAL)** does not provide an interest rate subsidy, and interest accrues over the entire loan period. Students may borrow up to $20,000 each year, up to a total of $80,000. Payments begin nine months after completing medical school. Deferments are granted for internship, residency, and/or military service. Since the rate of interest is the same as the interest on the 91-day Treasury bills plus three percent, it is variable.

The Federal Supplemental Loan to Students Program (SLS) is available to independent medical students who are ineligible to receive federal financing. Under this program, which has an interest rate that is not subsidized, the medical student may borrow up to $10,000 per year. Income is not a consideration for these loans, which are generally arranged by banks or credit unions.

Through the **AAMC MEDLOANS Program,** a student may apply for both a **Federal Stafford Loan** and the **Alternative Loan Program (ALP)** using the same form. The ALP, administered by the AAMC, has certain benefits for medical students. One of the most important is that it is nonneed-based. The total aggregate educational indebtedness of the student may not exceed $150,000 for the 1996–97 academic year.

Students may also obtain scholarships from a number of different sources. To begin, there are several federal scholarship programs. **The Scholarships for Disadvantaged Students Program** is available for medical students who have a disadvantaged background and significant financial need. As scholarships, they require no payback.

The Scholarship Program for Students With Exceptional Financial Need (EFN) pays up to the cost of tuition, books, and instruments, and a monthly living stipend. To be eligible for this program, students must demonstrate that they are essentially devoid of financial resources. Only one year of study will be covered.

Another scholarship program for students from financially disadvantaged backgrounds is the **Federal Assistance for Disadvantaged Health Professions Students Scholarship Program (FADHPS).** Though the amount of money available, which is dependent on federal allocations, varies from year to year, the scholarship may be used for tuition, fees, and other expenses.

Every state has a medical school financial aid program for its residents. For example, Massachusetts has state medical scholarships that are awarded to financially needy residents of the Commonwealth of Massachusetts. There are also private scholarship sources. Included in this list are the **Massachusetts State Federation of Women's Clubs Scholarship Programs,** that offers scholarships to female state residents, and the **Worcester Central District Medical Society,** which assists medical students from that area.

To obtain further information, contact the student assistance or higher educational authority in your state. And telephone your state and district medical societies to determine what scholarships they may have.

While some schools are better endowed than others, every medical school has certain endowment funds available for scholarships and loans. Thus, Johns Hopkins University School of Medicine has a wide array of financial assistance programs including scholarships, loans, and funding for research. For other schools the funding is far more limited.

Obviously, you should contact the medical school you will attend to discuss scholarship and loan opportunities. The vast majority of the funding you will receive will likely be obtained through the school's financial aid office. But there are other avenues.

In addition to federal scholarships and loans, I borrowed money, in the form of a no-interest loan, from the **Hattie M. Strong Foundation in Washington, D.C.** I repaid it a few years after graduation. The same foundation helped me secure funding for Jewish medical students through a bank in Pennsylvania. Although there was no obligation to repay the money, I felt that it would assist future medical students, and so I did.

You may be surprised to learn that there are a large number of private scholarships and loans available to only a small niche of medical students. Applicants must meet very specific requirements. Spend the time necessary to research these. They could prove to be an invaluable source.

By my third year of medical school, money was extremely tight. Since physicians were still subject to the draft, I knew that I had a two-year selective service obligation to complete. And, so, to fulfill my obligation and to help my financial situation, I decided to volunteer for the National Health Service Corps.

As a volunteer, I was allowed to complete medical school and internship. Then, I was sent to two different underserved areas for a total of two years of service. In return, during my fourth year of medical school, I was paid an ensign-level salary and received money for tuition and books.

These **National Health Service Corps Scholarships** are still available. In addition, similar scholarships may be obtained from the **Armed Forces Health Professions Scholarship Program.** Students who receive these monies are required to complete a certain amount of years in the National Health Service Corps or military.

I was also one of the earliest members of the **Commissioned Officer Student Training and Extern Program (COSTEP).** In the mid-60s, after my sophomore year of college, I was selected for this program. Beginning that summer, and continuing for the next four summers, I worked in laboratories at the National Institutes of Health in Bethesda, Maryland. The experience and the income proved invaluable. Unlike the National Health Service Corps, COSTEPs are not required to complete any post-graduation service. So those summers as a COSTEP never added to my selective service commitment. It is interesting to note, parenthetically, that it was as a COSTEP that I met fellow COSTEP Myrna Pauline Chandler, an undergraduate at Connecticut College, on July 8, 1969. Today, she is my wife, a journalist, and coauthor of this book.

Minority students should pay particular attention to the scholarships intended to serve minority populations. For example, there are scholarships specifically targeted for students of Chinese, Mexican, or Native American descent. **The Commonwealth Fund** assists academically-talented medical students who are minorities. Candidates generally are selected by the medical school. **The National Medical Fellowships** are another example of scholarships for minority students. And the **National Institute of Health** has summer research fellowships for first- and second-year minority medical students.

Minority applicants should carefully review the reference material. Contact programs directly. Also, you should work with the minority student program of your future medical school to see if it may be of any assistance.

Female medical students should be aware that there are many scholarships and loan programs specifically for women. There are loans from the **American Medical Women's Association Loan Program,** and financial assistance from the **American Association of University Women. The Daughters of the American Revolution** has programs, as does the **Business and Professional Women's Foundation.** Take the time to look into these and others. You never can tell which one could help you pay your way through medical school.

In this chapter I have presented only the briefest introduction to financing a medical education. Please use my information as a stepping stone. There are entire books on the topic. Local libraries and bookstores have many sources.

If you truly want to attend medical school and are accepted, do not let your lack of financial resources cause you to hesitate. Yes, it will be necessary to devote a portion of your time to applying for aid. And, yes, there will be sacrifices to be made. But the rewards are well worth the effort. Never let money, or the lack of it, stand between you and your dream.

References — Chapter Twelve

1. *Medical School Admission Requirements 1996–1997,* Association of American Medical Colleges, 1995.
2. *Financial Planning and Management Manual for U.S. Medical Students,* Association of American Medical Colleges.
3. Dennis, M.J., *Guide to Financing a Medical School Education,* 2nd Edition, Barron's, 1994.
4. *Minority School Opportunities in United States Medical Schools, 1994–95,* Association of American Medical Colleges, 1993.
5. Rothman E., "The Squeeze Is On," *Focus,* November 17, 1995.

Chapter Thirteen
. . . .

REJECTION

You thought you did everything right. You worked hard to earn good grades. You scored reasonably well on the MCATs. Your letters of reference showed you to be a solid candidate. Your extracurricular activities demonstrated leadership. And you were even invited for a few interviews. Yet, you were rejected by every single medical school to which you submitted an application.

Clearly you were up against staggering odds! For the class entering medical school in 1989 almost 27,000 students applied for 16,000 spaces; for the class entering medical school in 1995, there were approximately 47,000 individuals applying for slightly more than 16,000 spaces. Two out of every three applicants to medical school are rejected. In just a few years, the situation has become extremely competitive.

You may be disappointed

if you fail, but you're

doomed if you don't try."

Beverly Sills

So what do you do now? As soon as possible, notify your premedical advisor. Arrange to meet. Together, critically review any areas that might have led to your rejection. Talk about your timing of the application, your credentials, your letters of reference, and coursework. Very often, this critical review will shed light on one or more correctable weaknesses in your application. For example, some applicants apply later in the season after many of the medical schools have made the majority of their selections. Perhaps a grade in an important required premedical course might have been well below the standard. That may be corrected by taking another related course and earning an excellent grade. It is also possible that a letter of reference mentioned several shortcomings.

If you never were invited for any interviews, there is a good chance that your application had some serious difficulties. You and your advisor should attempt to determine if your application is able to be strengthened or whether the time has arrived to begin planning for another career.

I have been fortunate to have had a large number of outstanding premedical advisees. During the past three years, all of my advisees have been admitted to one or more U.S. medical school. In previous years, the vast majority of my advisees have been accepted. Only a very few were rejected. In one particular case, the advisee applied to both medical and dental school. Though he was rejected by medical schools, he was admitted to dental school. In another instance, a very well qualified candidate was rejected from numerous medical schools. She decided to spend some time working in a research laboratory. Two years later, she reapplied and was admitted to at least two U.S. medical schools.

Often there is an obvious reason why medical schools reject otherwise qualified candidates. Occasionally, there is no clear, causal factor. If you are truly interested in a medical career, and after discussions with your premedical advisor you wish to make an another attempt, you may be interested in statistics on reapplications to U.S. medical schools from 1983 through 1986 gathered by Paul Jolly, Ph.D., Associate Vice President for Operational studies of the Association of American Medical Colleges.

When Dr. Jolly reviewed 4,025 applicants who went on to reapply to medical school in 1986 after being rejected in 1985, he found 1,891 or 47 percent were admitted the second time around. Of the 1,583 applicants who reapplied in 1986 after being rejected in 1982, 1983, or 1984, 638 or 40.3 percent were accepted. Among those 1,704 applicants who had been rejected from medical school on two or three occasions, 681 or 40 percent were accepted. Interestingly, of all the first-time applicants in 1986, 13,310 or 57.5 percent were accepted.

Undoubtedly, an individual's best chance for admission to medical school is during the first round of applications. That is when you should make every effort to have an outstanding application. But if you have been rejected, the statistics indicate that reapplicants have a chance and do obtain admission.

If you do decide to reapply, you and your advisor must take the time to find the weaknesses in your first application. You must become involved in some type of meaningful work that will demonstrate you abilities and capabilities. Some students pursue further coursework or another degree such as a master's in science or public health. Others devote their energies to public service or medical research. Without demonstrating initiative, your chances for admission are markedly reduced.

Maintain contact with your premedical advisor. When it is time to reapply to medical school, your advisor will again prove to be an invaluable resource. Having the same advisor will show consistency, and add strength to your application.

Let's assume that you are eventually accepted to medical school. There are two interesting studies of the performance of medical students who were initially rejected by medical school. In the mid-1980s, Richard A. DeVaul, M.D., with the Office of Student Affairs of the University of Texas Medical School at Houston, *et. al.,* had a unique opportunity to investigate the subject. According to DeVaul, "In April 1979, the state legislature required that the class size of 150 be increased to 200 first-year students in September 1979. . . . The Admissions Committee therefore was asked in mid-May to select an additional 50 students from those applicants who were previously interviewed but not chosen. Of the cohort thus selected, 43 (86 percent) had not been accepted by any medical school as of May 1."

The researchers attempted to determine if there were any differences in medical school performance and attrition between these two groups and to locate academic or demographic variables common to the group that was first accepted. In order to compare the academic performance of the two groups, the researchers surveyed the students' preclinical grades from 22 courses and assessments of attending physicians and residents in the clinical clerkships. Scores on the National Board of Medical Examiners Part I and evaluations from residency program directors were also included.

> *If you want the present to be different from the past, study the past.*
>
> **Baruch Spinoza**

There were no significant differences in academic performance between the initially accepted group of 150 students and the 50 previously rejected students. Incredibly, only 28 percent of the differences between the two groups was the result of objective variables such as GPA and MCAT scores. The majority of variance between the two groups — a whopping 72 percent — appeared to be the direct result of the "subjective impression created" during the premedical interviewing process. This study seems to under score the pivotal role that the interview plays in admission.

As you rethink the medical school application process, try to review your interviews. Think of ways they might have been improved. Practice with friends and your premedical advisor. Read books on the topic.

James R. Jackson, Ph.D., Assistant Professor, Office of Educational Development, University of Alabama School of Medicine, *et. al.,* compared the academic performance of first-time applicants to reapplicants who entered the University of Alabama School of Medicine between 1978 and 1984. Of the students, 681 were first-time applicants and 399 applied two or more times. The researchers determined that "the reapplicants had lower preadmission measures and a higher rate of academic difficulty during medical school."

Nevertheless, the authors conclude that "reapplicants should not be viewed negatively simply because they are reapplicants." Moreover, "the process of reapplication reflects a certain amount of dedication and motivation." And admissions committees may be impressed by reapplicants who "take additional coursework or seek additional degrees."

Unfortunately, it is crucial to underscore the fact that the majority of reapplicants will not be accepted to medical school. Now you must decide. Are you truly dedicated to a career as a physician? Do you want to keep reapplying to medical schools, always facing the possibility of more rejections? Or, has the time arrived to begin to consider an alternative career? Only you may answer those questions.

Some rejected applicants select a profession that is related to their majors in college. Others enter public health or medical research. A few enter corresponding fields such as dentistry, physical therapy, or psychology.

Despite rejection, some people know that their true calling may be found in medicine. For those, there are two possibilities to consider.

In the 1970s, one of my relatives received only rejections from the numerous U.S medical schools to which he applied. Determined to pursue a career in medicine, he enrolled in a European medical school for two years and then successfully transferred to a U.S. medical school. After medical school, he completed an accredited U.S. residency program. Today, he is physician with a very active private practice.

Over the years, the rules have changed. It is no longer quite so easy to begin medical school in another country and then transfer to one in the U.S. Though it is not an impossible situation, there are more constraints. If you wish to attend a medical school in another country consider the following:

- With regard to academic quality, foreign medical schools rank from the outstanding to poor. Naturally, the quality of education you receive will impact your ability to pass any of the required U.S. examinations. Talk with friends, your premedical advisor, and physicians. Ask their opinions. Read reports such as *The Gourman Report.* Medical schools in Western Europe and North America are rated the highest.

- Language may be a problem. Are classes taught in English? If not, what is the language that is used? Are you fluent in that language?
- Then there is the cost. Assume that no financial aid will be available for U.S. citizens.
- Will distance from your family be a concern? Medical school years are difficult emotionally. How will you feel so far away from your familial ties?
- Are the people in the foreign country generally friendly to U.S. citizens? Would that impact on your ability to study and function?

Students who attend foreign medical schools often find it more difficult to obtain accredited residencies in the U.S. And they may not be as well prepared for the required examinations. But for those who, despite rejection, remain absolutely determined to become physicians, foreign medical schools may offer a possible alternative route.

Another choice may be to apply to colleges of osteopathic medicine. No newcomer to healing, osteopathic medicine was developed about 120 years ago by Andrew Taylor Still, M.D., a physician dissatisfied with the 19th century practice of medicine.

Osteopathic physicians (D.O.'s) pay particular attention to the musculoskeletal system which, they believe, reflects and influences the condition of all other body systems. In many ways, D.O. training is very similar to M.D. preparation. For example, to become a D.O. one must receive four years of undergraduate education followed by four more years of basic medical instruction. Those four years are typically followed by two to six years of residency. Like M.D.'s, D.O.'s may specialize in areas such as psychiatry, obstetrics, and surgery. They are required to pass state licensing examinations and are fully licensed to practice in a variety of settings.

Those who do not grow,

. . . .

grow smaller.

Rabbi Hillel, Talmud: Pirke Avot

According to the American Osteopathic Association (AOA), there are 15 accredited U.S. colleges of osteopathic medicine. Additionally, there is a college with provisional accreditation and another one in a preaccreditation state. The colleges are located in Florida,

California, Illinois, Missouri, Pennsylvania, Michigan, New York, Ohio, Oklahoma, New Jersey, Maine, Texas, Iowa, and West Virginia. During the academic year 1994–95, there were 7,600 osteopathic students and 36,561 doctors of osteopathy. Further, there were 153 internship training programs, 2,223 internship positions, 467 residency training programs, and 3,469 residency positions.

The American Osteopathic Association has certifying boards in a number of specialties, and in 1994 there were 10,285 board certified doctors of osteopathy. Doctors of osteopathy are fully trained and licensed to prescribe medications and to perform surgery. Most, however, work in family-oriented primary care practices, frequently in small towns and rural areas. The AOA contends that osteopathic physicians are known for their "whole person approach" to medicine, and they "focus on preventive health care." Osteopathic practice includes osteopathic manipulative treatment (OMT). "With OMT, osteopathic physicians use their hands to diagnose injury and illness and to encourage your body's natural tendency toward good health. By combining all other medical procedures with OMT, D.O.'s offer their patients the most comprehensive care available in medicine today."

An example of a school of osteopathy is the New York College of Osteopathic Medicine founded in 1977 and located in Old Westbury, New York. It offers a four-year, fully accredited program leading to the degree of Doctor of Osteopathy (D.O.).

The first two years of osteopathic education appear very similar to those of M.D. education. During the first year, however, there are also courses entitled Microanatomy (Histology) and Osteology, Principles of Osteopathic Manipulative Medicine, and the Application of Osteopathic Principles. The second year includes more advanced courses in osteopathy.

Though Osteopathic Manipulative Medicine is part of the third year curriculum, the major clinical clerkships are in medicine, surgery, family practice, obstetrics/gynecology, pediatrics, and psychiatry. The fourth year coursework is hospital-based and office-based primary care, emergency medicine, primary care selectives, specialty selectives, radiology, sub-internship, and electives.

Coursework during the first two years is on the college's campus. Training in the clinical sciences is on campus as well as at 14 affiliated hospitals, physicians' offices, and health centers. Following graduation, internship programs are available at the affiliated hospitals.

Remember, first time rejection from medical school may not signal the end of your career. You may wish to reapply, to contemplate study abroad, or investigate osteopathy. There are other choices. Sometimes it is necessary to take a few detours before the correct route is found.

References — Chapter Thirteen

1. *Medical School Admission Requirements 1996–1997,* Association of American Medical Colleges, 1995.
2. Jolly, P., "Datagram," *Journal of Medical Education,* 62:357–359, 1987.
3. Devaul, R.A., Jervey, F., Chappell, J.A., Caver, P., Short, B., O'Keefe, S., "Medical School Performance of Initially Rejected Applicants," *JAMA,* 257:47–51, 1987.
4. Jackson, J.R., Brooks, C.M., Brown, S., Scott, C.W., "Academic Performance of Reapplicants to a Medical School," *Academic Medicine,* 64:219–220, 1989.
5. *Catalog 1994–95,* New York College of Osteopathic Medicine, 1994.

Chapter Fourteen

. . . .

TIMETABLE

The previous 13 chapters have outlined the process of applying to medical school. If you are a middle or high school student who is already planning a career in medicine, it is not too early to take specific actions that may one day help your application. Consider volunteering or applying for internships in the health care field. And work hard to maintain a very strong academic average. For further ideas review Table 14-1.

Table 14-2 provides a timetable for the first two and three-quarter years of college, concluding with the recommendation that the Medical College Admission Test (MCAT) be taken in April of the junior year.

The last table, Table 14-3, outlines the 17 months prior to matriculation at your chosen medical school. This is the period of greatest intensity. While there may be variations in the timetable, after years of working in the field I have found this one to be the most effective. And it should provide the premedical student with the sequence of events necessary for admission to medical school. Although I've said it before, it is worth repeating — **Your application must be submitted in a timely manner. A late application significantly reduces chances for admission.**

The door of success is marked "push" and "pull."

Achieving success is knowing when to do what.

Yiddish Folk Saying

To glean an even better sense of a medical school, my premedical advisees often like to meet with medical students. That is why I have asked one of my former students to write about her experiences at Harvard Medical School. This book will end with her comments.

The medicine I currently practice and teach is not what I studied in school. Over the years, the practice of medicine has undergone rapid transformations. Today, that change is happening at an even faster pace. Managed care, a term I never heard in medical school, is now utilized by increasing percentages of people in the U.S.

Table 14-1
Timetable for Middle and High School Students

Middle school years	Consider career choices
10th Grade	Volunteer in local hospitals, nursing homes
11th Grade	Seek opportunities to work in a health or biomedical field
12th Grade	Gain acceptance to the college of your choice. Consider combined baccalaureate/M.D.

Table 14-2
Timetable for First Two and Three-Quarter Years of College

First year	Work very hard, take premed courses, participate in extracurricular activities, enjoy college
Summer	Travel, seek research or human service position
Second year, first term	Make contact with premed office
Second year, second term	First meeting with premed advisor, introductions
Summer	Volunteer in hospital, research, or medically related position
October/November	Meet with advisor, review application, activities, grades, courses
February	Meet with advisor, begin to firm up letter, discuss MCAT, AMCAS, study for MCAT
April	Take MCAT

Due to the advent of expensive technological procedures and the proliferation of subspecialists, the cost of medical care is escalating at an alarming rate.

It is also fair to say that in certain areas of the U.S. there is an overabundance of subspecialists. At the same time, in other sections of the country, there are shortages of primary care physicians. Many experts in the field have suggested that there will be greater

Table 14-3
Timetable for Last 17 Months of College

April	Take MCAT, write to schools for information
May	Work with advisor on school list
June	Work on personal statement
July	Compete and submit AMCAS
August	Early decision applications due. Be certain letters of recommendation are complete
September	Complete secondaries
October	Early decision applicants notified, meet with advisor, practice interview
October through April	Interviews, acceptances, financial aid applications
May 15	Select one school
June through August	May hear from wait-listed schools
August/September	Matriculation!

demands for the generalists or primary care physicians. Some believe that medical schools use various means to encourage more students to enter primary care and will accept more students who indicate a strong interest in primary care.

It is significant to mention that for the first time in recent years, in 1995, the National Resident Matching Program matched over half of the 13,549 U.S. medical school fourth year students to internships in primary care. Fifty-one percent of the nation's new interns selected training in one of the generalists disciplines — family practice, internal medicine, or pediatrics. There is increasing demand for well trained primary care physicains.

I don't think of all the misery, but of all the beauty that still remains.

Anne Frank

However, there are stories of anesthesiologists or eye surgeons or neurosurgeons who are unable to secure a good position in their selected specialty. It was reported that an anesthesia residency program in New York will reduce the number of residents over the next several years. In 1995, there was a decline in students matched to programs in radiology and anesthesiology.

I have never regretted my decision to become a physician. Despite all the negative publicity that the field occasionally receives — the abusive practices of unethical providers, the administration of an incorrect medicine, or the frequency of unnecessary or inappropriate surgery, I am as convinced today as I was more than three decades ago that medicine is one of the finest careers. Nothing is more exciting than working with and helping patients. Over and over again, after caring for children and adolescents, I have been able to experience the thanks and satisfaction of family members. And it is no exaggeration to say that as a physician one may work at the cutting edge of technology. Future research promises even more exciting advances.

For those who wish, a career in medicine offers boundless challenges and opportunities. The art and science of medicine may not be duplicated by any other career choice.

References — Chapter Fourteen

1. Rosenthal, E., "Young Doctors Find Specialist Jobs Hard to Get," *New York Times,* April 15, 1995.
2. Eichna, L.W., "Medical School Education, 1975–1979, *NEJM,* 303:727–734, 1980.

Chapter Fifteen
. . . .

EPILOGUE – THE MEDICAL SCHOOL EXPERIENCE: A PERSONAL PERSPECTIVE

Eva Chittenden, M.D.

Dr. Chittenden graduated from Harvard Medical School in June 1995. She began her residency in medicine at the Beth Israel Hospital, Boston, in July 1995. Although she was not my premedical advisee, she was my student for one year in a longitudinal course in Adolescent Medicine at the Boston Children's Hospital. She provides valuable insight into the medical school experience.

I went to medical school without having truly decided that I wanted to be a doctor. I had thought about other careers such as law, public policy, and public health. I didn't know what it was like to be a medical student or a doctor, even though I had done the prerequisites: talked with medical students, visited their classes, shadowed doctors, worked as a medical research assistant, and read books about medical school (some of which, incidentally, almost convinced me **not** to go to medical school).

I had not had the inside view that one gets by having a doctor for a parent; nor had I had any physician role models growing up. As a result, I was worried. How did I know this would be right for me? How did I know that I would like being a doctor? The fact is I didn't know and couldn't know, but nonetheless had to make a decision.

One important factor was the realization that medicine opened up numerous career paths — from clinical work to teaching to research to public policy — and that odds were that I would find a niche. More importantly, I felt that medicine suited my personality better than law. I was more comfortable with the image of myself as caregiver and nurturer than as debater or adversary. I liked to work with others and knew that medicine required team work. I entered medical school promising myself that I could leave after a year if I were unhappy. I am incredibly glad I went; it was the best decision I ever made.

First year was an absorbing, and at times, disorienting experience. I was entering a new world with a new language: "patella, alveolus, neutrophil, countercurrent mechanism." I remember sitting in small group discussion feeling utterly lost. Conversation flowed around me and I only caught bits and pieces. I wondered if I was less intelligent than my classmates and then lost even further touch with the conversation. I recall looking into my microscope and seeing nothing but clouds until my professor came over and showed me how to focus the scope. In lecture, biochemical pathways flew right over my head. Kidney physiology entered my ears but did not synapse with neurons in my brain. I panicked before tests. I worried I would fail and studied intensely. I longed for the days in college when I had a sense of mastery over a subject, when I could wrap my mind around a manageable amount of material and excel on exams.

Anatomy lab was a foreign land within a foreign world. Most of the time, dissecting a cadaver was an interesting academic exercise. I concentrated on the origins and insertions of muscles and on the pathways of arteries and nerves. I was alternatively bored and fascinated by the complexity of the human body. I hated the smell of the formaldehyde used to preserve the bodies. The smell infiltrated my clothes and I quickly returned to the dorm to shower after each session. At times, however, I would snap out of my intellectual reverie and be flooded with uneasy questions. Who had this person been? Like me, this person had been alive and unique, and like him, I would be dead one day. How could I be so detached and see only a body? Would I be able to be so generous with my body when I died? I sometimes imagined that we were participating in a violent act, a dark primitive ritual of some kind, rather than a vital learning experience. Unlike some of my classmates, I was unable to return to the lab at night for further exploring. At some level, the experience brought back childhood fears of death and ghosts. Fortunately, I was able to appreciate the importance and depth of this learning experience as well as the amazing gift I had been given by a stranger.

During the first year, I found classmates who felt similarly about these formative experiences. Sharing our feelings became a wonderful source of support and foundation for friendships. Not only did I make new friends, but I realized that I wasn't alone in feeling stupid and overwhelmed in class. Other students had been humanities majors in college and were struggling with the basic sciences. In addition, I found that many of my classmates also struggled with the many layers of meanings in dissecting cadavers.

Second year was more of first year with some important changes. I felt more comfortable in small group discussions and spoke out more. The subject matter was more interesting. Seemingly abstract biochemical pathways were replaced by the pathophysiology of diseases we would see in people. Learning how to examine patients, however, was once again entering completely new territory. We showed up at our respective hospitals with our white coats and doctors' bags, feeling like impostors. I felt relieved that my name tag said "medical student." I didn't want to pretend I was anything other than I was. After practicing the physical exam on one another, we practiced on patients. As the year went on, we each spent a few hours a week with a patient, laboriously taking a history and then fumbling through the physical exam. Although the patients had agreed to participate and although I went out of my way to be courteous and sympathetic to their plight (both their illness and their having to put up with me), I still felt like an intruder. A few times, I was asked to leave prematurely. The patient, understandably, had become impatient or fatigued. I felt incompetent and angry at the same time. I had always been good at things, so why wasn't I good at this? We had to learn to "present" to faculty, that is, to organize the patient's words and our physical exam findings into technical and precise medical language. This was a difficult but important skill. During one of my first presentations, I was stopped suddenly in midstream by my preceptor who told me that I was using "English" rather than medical language. She told me that a medical presentation "wasn't supposed to be in novel format." English and Spanish were the only languages I knew, I wanted to tell her angrily as tears welled up in my eyes.

Second year had its lighter moments. For a month in the middle of the year, classes took a back seat to rehearsals as we prepared for our second year show, a wonderful forum for us to display our myriad nonmedical talents — writing, directing, singing, dancing, and acting. I discovered that my lab partner had a wonderful voice and that a friend was a closet electric guitarist. I danced as a hippie, a 1950s school girl, and a macrophage. It was a time for the class to bond before we dispersed among the hospitals. I was also able to choose from a variety of extracurricular activities. I helped raise money and plan activities for the "Czech Project," a cultural exchange between Czech and U.S. medical students. A group of us hosted 15 Czech students, introducing them to life and medicine in the U.S. We then traveled to Prague for the second half of the exchange.

The last months of second year were perhaps the worst time in medical school. While anticipating third year (when we would leave the classroom behind for bedside teaching) with both excitement and fear, we were cramming innumerable details into our brains in preparation for the first part of the National Boards, a two-day extravaganza of multiple choice questions. Although the exam was an opportunity to synthesize the material of the first two years, it was another experience which challenged my ego. When I found myself guessing on question after question, how could I help but wonder what I had been doing the first two years. Had I been having too much fun? Was I just stupid? The antidote, as always, was sharing my experience with friends and realizing I wasn't alone. Like all my friends, I came out on the other side having done just fine on the exam.

The first two years of medical school were an opportunity to redefine my priorities. For much of my life, I had put incredible pressure on myself to excel. And although I had succeeded, it had been at a cost. In high school, I sacrificed a social life. My time was spent studying or in ballet class, pursuing my dream to be a dancer. In college, I succeeded at the cost of finding pleasure in my work. Writing papers and taking exams made me anxious because I had such high expectations of myself. In medical school, I consciously decided to work hard, but not to expect perfection. I was determined to find time for other activities — time with friends, dance performances, swimming, yoga, and reading. I took courses which broadened my view of medicine, including the History of Medicine and Medicine & Literature. Although I felt less prepared for classes and for third year, it was a worthwhile trade-off. I learned to accept my lack of knowledge, a feeling we all have to accept as doctors. I can also say that I enjoyed the first two years of medical school. Instead of feeling burned out by intense studying, I looked forward to learning more. Moreover, I had the conviction that being a good doctor meant not only having the most up-to-date knowledge but also being available emotionally to patients. And, to do this, I felt I had to take care of myself.

In the third year, we made the dramatic transition from classroom to hospital. We spent our time "rotating" through the various hospitals and services, including internal medicine, pediatrics, surgery, and obstetrics and gynecology. We admitted and cared for patients under the supervision of housestaff (interns and residents) and "presented" our patients to faculty in Teaching Rounds. Like the housestaff, we spent nights in the hospital "on call." Though we had spent some time in the hospital during the first two years, the hospital was still an alien place. Given my apprehensions, I decided to ease into third year, starting with the relatively "benign" rotations, psychiatry, and radiology. My roommate jumped right in, starting off with internal medicine. She described the experience as "struggling to keep her nose above water." She borrowed the metaphor from the course director who had told the students to expect a smooth transition from "nose above water" to dry land during the first month of the rotation. Many of us experienced a slower and bumpier transition. While we occasionally made it onto land, we often fell back into the water to be submerged again.

In the hospital, the skills necessary to succeed were quite different from those of the first two years. The ability to work as a team member, to be enthusiastic and to figure out when to ask questions and when to be quiet were all important skills. These social skills were as important as depth of knowledge. Hiding feelings of anger or disappointment when we were ignored or treated badly was critical; interns and residents were already under a great deal of stress themselves. There was a machismo to the environment and we were expected to put up with a certain amount of abuse. On the positive note, the ability to communicate and empathize with patients was recognized. Although I still struggled with feelings of insecurity and was forced to confront the unpleasant realities of sleep deprivation and low status, I felt more in my element. I was excited to be finally caring for patients and received positive feedback on my interpersonal skills from both patients and faculty. When I was discouraged, spending extra time talking with patients allowed me to feel better about myself and put my own feelings into perspective.

There were many formative experiences. Delivering a baby, scrubbing in for surgery, seeing a gun-shot victim, and watching a patient in a near-death breathing rhythm were rites of passage which reminded me of standing in toe shoes for the first time in ballet class. There were the quieter, but equally privileged moments, of sitting with patients while they shared private concerns and anxieties. Our position as medical students was unique; we weren't yet doctors, but neither were we patients. Like patients, however, we often felt a loss of control. This position of partial outsider allowed us to empathize more easily with patients. One night during my internal medicine rotation, I admitted a 40-year-old man with AIDS who had intractable abdominal pain and diarrhea. The patient was discouraged and angry and had difficulty cooperating with our team. In the hospital the inevitable "work-up" began as a series of increasingly invasive diagnostic tests were initiated. The patient became angrier by the hour. When I sat down with him, he told me that he wanted to go home because "he was tired and had had enough pushing, poking, and prodding." He refused further tests. Although I relayed his wishes to my intern and resident, they pursued the work-up aggressively with the hope of finding a diagnosis. Four days into his stay, the patient announced his intention to leave and ignore treatment. It was wrenching to watch him attempt to put on his clothes, a previously simple act which he could no longer perform independently. I pleaded with him to continue his care as an outpatient. Even though he and the residents were able to work out their differences — he agreed to return for care — I was left with many uncomfortable feelings. Why hadn't they taken the time to listen to the man's wishes from the beginning and why hadn't they respected his wishes once they became clear? The residents seemed determined to go to every length to fight the man's illness, making it their battle rather than the patient's.

Midway through the third year, I decided to take a year away from school. I didn't feel ready to go on to the fourth year. While I knew I wanted to be a doctor, I hadn't decided on a specialty. I was considering internal medicine, pediatrics, and psychiatry. Third year is a difficult time to make this important decision because one has so little time and energy to reflect on one's experiences and to explore the options. I had another agenda as well. I wanted to strengthen my fund of knowledge. During the third year, I had been praised for my interpersonal skills but had also been told that my knowledge base was weak. Though I was assured that I would catch up and that other students often received this feedback, I wasn't so sure. Since I was often worried about my performance on the wards, I found it hard to distance myself enough to imagine my future as a doctor, much less as a specific kind of doctor.

At Harvard, taking a year away from medical school was not only acceptable but encouraged. A sizeable minority of a class chooses to do this each year. Activities range from clinical or lab research to overseas medical projects to starting a rock band to studying cooking in France. I designed my year to fit my needs. I obtained a pathology fellowship from one of the Harvard hospitals as a way to revisit pathophysiology from a different angle and thus reinforce my medical knowledge. In the first half of the year, I rotated through various fields of pathology. While assisting with autopsies, I developed a visual and tactile feeling for the effects of disease on various organs. I then viewed these same effects under the microscope (which I could now focus). I reviewed microbiology and hematology in the clinical labs. The second half of the year was set aside for lab research. Although I learned a great deal from my project, both about neuropathology and the process of research, I discovered that lab research was not for me. I missed patient care.

I also spent one evening a week at a clinic at Children's Hospital seeing teenagers with an adolescent specialist. During this pivotal time, I began to feel like a physician and to leave my self doubts behind. Over the year, I built up a small panel of patients who saw me as their doctor. I became interested in their lives and in the issues they faced growing up in the inner city: sexually transmitted disease, teenage pregnancy, poverty, violence, and depression. I also found a mentor in the physician with whom I worked, an unusual opportunity in medical school given that we change rotations each month. To my relief, I found a kind of medicine that I could see myself pursuing. I would become a doctor who knew my patients well, and over time, who was interested in patients as people, and who would pay close attention to social contexts and their effect on health.

During the year, I had another opportunity. Harvard had just begun a program in which fourth year students assisted in teaching the second year physical exam course. For the first time in medical school, I realized how much I knew and enjoyed sharing this knowledge with others. The experiences in the Adolescent Clinic and in the physical exam course stimulated my interests in primary care medicine and teaching. The pathology fellowship enabled me to enter fourth year with renewed confidence in my medical knowledge.

Fourth year is a mix of more hospital rotations, both required and elective, and of negotiating the eight-month process of applying for residency. While I still had my ups and downs in the hospital (and will inevitably continue to have them during residency), I was more comfortable. Now more skilled and independent, I no longer increased the intern's work loads. Because I was more relaxed, I enjoyed my interactions with housestaff, attendings, and patients more, and I began to appreciate the intellectual challenges of medicine. I liked being asked to defend a diagnostic test or treatment I had proposed or to do a presentation on relevant literature.

I felt better equipped to understand the feelings of my patients and their families, as well as the feelings these generated in me.

During a month in the intensive care unit, I helped care for a healthy young woman who had become seriously ill after a routine operation. The photos on the wall showed a vibrant woman with her husband and three young children which one could not help but contrast with the unconscious patient connected to machines. When I saw the exhaustion and profound grief on her husband's face, I felt very sad. My sadness, I believe, allowed me to connect better with the husband as we discussed her condition. Many people say that as medical students we must learn to protect ourselves from the overwhelming feelings generated by patients' suffering without becoming too detached. I am sure this is true for many of us. The process I went through, however, was almost the inverse. The high expectations I had placed on myself (and others had placed on me) during my life had made me somewhat self-absorbed. To excel in a high-powered world, I had to look out for my own interests. Looking back, I think I was somewhat detached from patients at the start of medical school. As I gained more confidence in the hospital and clinic, I became more able to feel for patients and their families. And far from threatening my own stability, this only made my work more rewarding.

While fourth year ends with graduation, its most dramatic moment occurs in mid-March on "Match Day." All across the country, medical students are simultaneously handed envelopes containing their hospital assignments for residency — our postgraduate training. It is a moment of high drama. Some of us rejoice and some of us are disappointed. It is the culmination of an eight-month application process. For me, choosing a specialty was more difficult than the process of applying. By the fall of fourth year, I was still debating between internal medicine and combined training in medicine and pediatrics. And I had not entirely excluded psychiatry. Just as I had done prior to medical school, I talked with many people, looked inside myself, and then of course decided. I had to accept that there was no right answer and that I would probably be happy in any of these fields. I chose internal medicine because medicine-pediatrics felt too broad and because, when I really thought about it, I preferred working with adults. I'll always wonder about psychiatry. But I realized that I would see many patients with psychiatric illness in a general medicine practice. Match Day, however, had meanings beyond finding out which hospital would be my home in the coming years. It was a time to look beyond medical school and to begin to internalize the image of myself as a doctor. I began to look forward with excitement to having my own patients, signing my own orders, and finally receiving a paycheck.

My classmates and I came to medical school with diverse interests and backgrounds, and we all participated in the same demanding and rigorous process which molded us into doctors. Toward the end of this shaping process, we became more comfortable with our skills and identities as physicians. We then watched our individual voices emerge in our work with patients and colleagues. In my mind, this process of professionalization is similar to that of becoming a dancer. For years on end, an aspiring ballerina must hone her technique and mold her body into a specific and pre-defined form. However, to complete her transformation into dancer, she must bring her unique personality and style to her dancing. By the end of medical school, we have hopefully begun our transformation into physicians with unique personalities and styles.

Medical school has been a difficult but rewarding journey for me. But it is only the beginning of the lifelong journey of being a doctor. Five years ago, I entered a new world hesitantly, unsure of myself and my footing. Now I have a new language, a new-found confidence, and a feeling of excitement and anticipation. Nothing is static in medicine. As doctors, we have endless opportunities to grow. We can learn about new medical advances daily, and we can also learn from each patient what it means to live in a particular culture and social situation and to struggle with life, illness, and death. If we allow them to, patients give us the opportunity to look inside ourselves. In one month I will graduate and become a doctor. I feel extraordinarily blessed.

Appendix I
· · · · · · · ·

UNITED STATES
MEDICAL SCHOOLS

Alabama
Office of Medical Student Services/
  Admissions
University of Alabama School of
  Medicine
VH100
Birmingham, Alabama 32594-0019
(205) 934-2330; FAX (205) 934-8724

Office of Admissions
Room 2015, Medical Sciences Building
University of South Alabama College
  of Medicine
Mobile, Alabama 36688
(334) 460-7176; FAX (334) 460-6278

Arizona
Admissions Office
University of Arizona College of
  Medicine
Tucson, Arizona 85724
(602) 626-6214; FAX (602) 626-4884

Arkansas
Office of Student Admissions, Slot 551
University of Arkansas for Medical
  Sciences
College of Medicine
4301 West Markham Street
Little Rock, Arkansas 72205
(501) 686-5354; FAX (501) 686-5873

California
Admissions Office
University of California, Davis
School of Medicine
Davis, California 95616
(916) 752-2717

Office of Admissions
University of California, Irvine
College of Medicine
118 Med Surge I
Irvine, California 92717
(714) 824-5388; FAX (714) 824-2083

Office of Student Affairs
Division of Admissions
University of California, Los Angeles
School of Medicine
Center for Health Sciences
Los Angeles, California 90024-1720
(310) 825-6081

Office of Admissions, 0621
Medical Teaching Facility
University of California, San Diego
School of Medicine
9500 Gilman Drive
La Jolla, California 92093-0621
(619) 534-3880; FAX (619) 534-5282

School of Medicine, Admissions
C-200, Box 0408
University of California, San Francisco
San Francisco, California 94143
(415) 476-4044

Associate Dean for Admissions
Loma Linda University
School of Medicine
Loma Linda, California 92350
(909) 824-4467; FAX (909) 824-4146

Office of Admissions
University of Southern California
School of Medicine
1975 Zonal Avenue
Los Angeles, California 90033
(213) 342-2552

Office of Admissions
Stanford University School of Medicine
851 Welch Road-Room 154
Palo Alto, California 94304-1677
(415) 723-6861; FAX (415) 725-4599

Colorado

Medical School Admissions
University of Colorado
School of Medicine
4200 East 9th Avenue, C-292
Denver, Colorado 80262
(303) 270-7361; FAX (303) 270-8494

Connecticut

Office of Admissions and Student
  Affairs
University of Connecticut School
  of Medicine
University of Connecticut Health
  Center
263 Farmington Avenue, Room AG-062
Farmington, Connecticut 06032
(203) 679-2152; FAX (203) 679-1282

Office of Admissions
Yale University
School of Medicine
367 Cedar Street
New Haven, Connecticut 06510
(203) 785-2696; FAX (203) 785-3234

District of Columbia

Office of Admissions
George Washington University
School of Medicine and Health Sciences
2300 Eye Street, N.W.
Washington, D.C. 20037
(202) 994-3506

Office of Admissions
Georgetown University School
  of Medicine
3900 Reservoir Road, N.W.
Washington, D.C. 20007
(202) 687-1154

Admissions Office
Howard University College of Medicine
520 W Street, N.W.
Washington, D.C. 20059
(202) 806-6270; FAX (202) 806-7934

Florida

Chairman, Medical Selection
  Committee
Box 100216
J. Hillis Miller Health Center
University of Florida College of
  Medicine
Gainesville, Florida 32610
(904) 392-4569; FAX (904) 392-6482

Office of Admissions
University of Miami School of Medicine
P.O. Box 016159
Miami, Florida 33101
(305) 547-6791; FAX (305) 547-6548

Office of Admissions
Box 3
University of South Florida College
  of Medicine
12901 Bruce B. Downs Boulevard
Tampa, Florida 33612-4799
(813) 974-2229; FAX (813) 974-4990

Georgia

Medical School Admissions
Room 303, Woodruff Health Sciences
  Center
Administration Building
Emory University School of Medicine
Atlanta, Georgia 30322-4510
(404) 727-5660; FAX (404) 727-0045

Dr. Mary Ella Logan
Associate Dean for Admissions
School of Medicine
Medical College of Georgia
Augusta, Georgia 30912-4760
(706) 721-3186; FAX (706) 721-0959

Office of Admissions and Student
  Affairs
Mercer University School of Medicine
Macon, Georgia 31207
(912) 752-2542

Admissions and Student Affairs
Morehouse School of Medicine
720 Westview Drive, S.W.
Atlanta, Georgia 30310-1495
(404) 752-1650; (404) 752-1512

Hawaii

Office of Admissions
University of Hawaii
John A. Burns School of Medicine
1960 East-West Road
Honolulu, Hawaii 96822
(808) 956-5446; FAX (808) 956-9547

Illinois

Office of the Dean of Students
University of Chicago
Pritzker School of Medicine
Billings Hospital Room G-115A,
  MC-1139
5841 South Maryland Avenue
Chicago, Illinois 60637
(312) 702-1939; FAX (312) 702-2598

Office of Admissions
UHS/Chicago Medical School
3333 Green Bay Road
North Chicago, Illinois 60064
(708) 578-3206; FAX (708) 578-3284

Office of Medical College Admissions
Room 165 CME M/C 783
University of Illinois
College of Medicine
808 S. Wood Street
Chicago, Illinois 60612
(312) 996-5635; FAX (312) 996-6693

Office of Admissions, Room 1752
Loyola University Medical Center
Stritch School of Medicine
2160 South First Avenue
Maywood, Illinois 60153
(708) 216-3229

Associate Dean for Admissions
Northwestern University Medical
   School
303 East Chicago Avenue
Chicago, Illinois 60611
(312) 503-8206

Office of Admissions
524 Academic Facility
Rush Medical College of Rush
   University
600 South Paulina Street
Chicago, Illinois 60612
(312) 942-6913; FAX (312) 942-2333

Office of Student and Alumni Affairs
Southern Illinois University
School of Medicine
P.O. Box 19230
Springfield, Illinois 62794-9230
(217) 524-0326; FAX (217) 785-5538

Indiana
Medical School Admissions Office
Fesler Hall 213
Indiana University School of Medicine
1120 South Drive
Indianapolis, Indiana 46202-5113
(317) 274-3772

Iowa
Coordinator of Admissions
108 CMAB
University of Iowa College of Medicine
Iowa City, Iowa 52242
(319) 335-8052; FAX (319) 335-8049

Kansas
Associate Dean for Admissions
University of Kansas School of Medicine
3901 Rainbow Boulevard
Kansas City, Kansas 66160-7301
(913) 588-5245; FAX (913) 588-5259

Kentucky
Admissions, Room MN-104
Office of Education
University of Kentucky College
   of Medicine
Chandler Medical Center
800 Rose Street
Lexington, Kentucky 40536-0084
(606) 323-6161; FAX (606) 323-2076

Office of Admissions
School of Medicine
Health Sciences Center
University of Louisville
Louisville, Kentucky 40292
(502) 852-5193

Louisiana
Admissions Office
Louisiana State University
School of Medicine in New Orleans
1901 Perdid Street
New Orleans, Louisiana 70112-1393
(504) 568-6262; FAX (504) 568-7701

Office of Student Admissions
Louisiana State University Medical
   Center
School of Medicine in Shreveport
P.O. Box 33932
Shreveport, Louisiana 71130-3932
(318) 675-5190; FAX (318) 675-5244

Office of Admissions
Tulane University School of Medicine
1430 Tulane Avenue, SL67
New Orleans, Louisiana 70112-2699
(504) 588-5187

Maryland
Committee on Admission
Johns Hopkins University
School of Medicine
720 Rutland Avenue
Baltimore, Maryland 21205-2196
(410) 955-3182

Committee on Admissions
Room 1-005
University of Maryland School
   of Medicine
655 West Baltimore Street
Baltimore, Maryland 21201
(410) 706-7478

Admissions Office, Room A-1041
Uniformed Services University of the
   Health Sciences
F. Edward Hebert School of Medicine
4301 Jones Bridge Road
Bethesda, Maryland 20814-4799
(301) 295-3101; (800) 772-1743
FAX (301) 295-3545

Massachusetts

Admissions Office
Building L, Room 124
Boston University School of Medicine
80 East Concord Street
Boston, Massachusetts 02118
(617) 638-4630

Admissions Office
Harvard Medical School
25 Shattuck Street
Boston, Massachusetts 02115-6092
(617) 432-1550; FAX (617) 432-3307

Associate Dean for Student Admissions
University of Massachusetts Medical
  School
55 Lake Avenue, North
Worcester, Massachusetts 01655
(508) 856-2323

Office of Admissions
Tufts University School of Medicine
136 Harrison Avenue, Stearns I
Boston, Massachusetts 02111
(617) 636-6571

Michigan

College of Human Medicine
Office of Admissions
A-239 Life Sciences
Michigan State University
East Lansing, Michigan 48824-1317
(517) 353-9620; FAX (517) 432-1051

Admissions Office
M4130 Medical Science I Building
University of Michigan Medical School
Ann Arbor, Michigan 48109-0611
(313) 764-6317; FAX (313) 936-3510

Director of Admissions
Wayne State University
540 East Canfield
Detroit, Michigan 48201
(313) 577-1466

Minnesota

Admissions Committee
Mayo Medical School
200 First Avenue, S.W.
Rochester, Minnesota 55905
(507) 284-3671; FAX (507) 284-2634

Office of Admissions, Room 107
University of Minnesota-Duluth School
  of Medicine
10 University Drive
Duluth, Minnesota 55812
(218) 726-8511; FAX (218) 726-6235

Office of Admissions and Student
  Affairs
Box 293-UMHC
University of Minnesota Medical School
420 Delaware Street, S.E.
Minneapolis, Minnesota 55455-0310
(612) 624-1122; FAX (612) 626-6800

Mississippi

Chairman, Admissions Committee
University of Mississippi School
  of Medicine
2500 North State Street
Jackson, Mississippi 39216-4505
(601) 984-5010; FAX (601) 984-5008

Missouri

Office of Admissions
MA202 Medical Sciences Building
University of Missouri-Columbia
School of Medicine
One Hospital Drive
Columbia , Missouri 65212
(314) 882-2923; FAX (314) 884-4808

Council on Selection
University of Missouri-Kansas City
School of Medicine
2411 Holmes
Kansas City, Missouri 64108
(816) 235-1870; FAX (816) 235-5277

Ms. Nancy McPeters
Admissions Committee
Saint Louis University School
  of Medicine
1402 South Grand Boulevard
St. Louis, Missouri 63104
(314) 577-8205; FAX (314) 577-8214

Office of Admissions
Washington University School
  of Medicine
660 South Euclid Avenue #8107
St. Louis, Missouri 63110
(314) 362-6857; FAX (314) 362-4658

Nebraska

Office of Medical School Admissions
Creighton University School
  of Medicine
2500 California Plaza
Omaha, Nebraska 68178
(402) 280-2798; FAX (402) 280-1241

Office of Academic Affairs
University of Nebraska College
  of Medicine
Room 4004 Conkling Hall
600 South 42nd Street
Omaha, Nebraska 68198-4430
(402) 559-4205; FAX (402) 559-4104

Nevada

Office of Admissions and Student
Affairs
University of Nevada School
of Medicine
Mail Stop 357
Reno, Nevada 89557
(702) 784-6063; FAX (702) 784-6096

New Hampshire

Admissions
Dartmouth Medical School
7020 Remsen, Room 306
Hanover, New Hampshire 03755-3833
(603) 650-1505; FAX (603) 650-1614

New Jersey

Director of Admissions
UMDNJ-New Jersey Medical School
185 South Orange Avenue
Newark, New Jersey 07103
(201) 982-4631; FAX (201) 982-7986

Office of Admissions
UMDNJ-Robert Wood Johnson
Medical School
675 Hoes Lane
Piscataway, New Jersey 08854-5635
(908) 235-4576; FAX (908) 235-5078

New Mexico

Office of Admissions and Student
Affairs
University of New Mexico School
of Medicine
Basic Medical Sciences Building,
Room 107
Albuquerque, New Mexico 87131-5166
(505) 277-4766; FAX (505) 277-2755

New York

Office of Admissions, A-3
Albany Medical College
47 New Scotland Avenue
Albany, New York 12208
(518) 262-5521; FAX (518) 262-5887

Office of Admissions
Albert Einstein College of Medicine
of Yeshiva University
Jack and Pearl Resnick Campus
1300 Morris Park Avenue
Bronx, New York 10461
(718) 430-2106; FAX (718) 430-8825

Columbia University College
of Physicians and Surgeons
Admissions Office, Room 1-416
630 West 168th Street
New York, New York 10032
(212) 305-3595

Office of Admissions
Cornell University Medical College
445 East 69th Street
New York, New York 10021
(212) 746-1067

Director of Admissions
Mount Sinai School of Medicine
Annenberg Building, Room 5-04
One Gustave L. Levy Place-Box 1002
New York, New York 10029-6574
(212) 241-6696

Office of Admissions
Room 127, Sunshine Cottage
New York Medical College
Valhalla, New York 10595
(914) 993-4507

Office of Admissions
New York University School of Medicine
P.O. Box 1924
New York, New York 10016
(212) 263-5290

Director of Admissions
University of Rochester School
of Medicine and Dentistry
Medical Center Box 601
Rochester, New York 14642
(716) 275-4539; FAX (716) 273-1016

Director of Admissions
State University of New York
Health Science Center at Brooklyn
450 Clarkson Avenue-Box 60M
Brooklyn, New York 11203
(718) 270-2446

Office of Medical Admissions
State University of New York at Buffalo
CFS Building
Room 35
Buffalo, New York 14214-3013
(716) 829-3465

Committee on Admissions
Level 4, Room 147
Health Sciences Center
SUNY Stony Brook
School of Medicine
Stony Brook, New York 11794-8434
(516) 444-2113; FAX (516) 444-2202

Admissions Committee
State Universiy of New York
Health Science Center at Syracuse
College of Medicine
155 Elizabeth Blackwell Street
Syracuse, New York 13210
(315) 464-4570; FAX (315) 464-8867

North Carolina

Office of Medical School Admissions
Bowman Gray School of Medicine
of Wake Forest University
Medical Center Boulevard
Winston-Salem, North Carolina
27157-1090
(910) 716-4264; FAX (910) 716-5807

Committee on Admissions
Duke University School of Medicine
Duke University Medical Center
P.O. Box 3710
Durham, North Carolina 27710
(919) 684-2985; FAX (919) 684-8893

Associate Dean
Office of Admissions
East Carolina University School
of Medicine
Greenville, North Carolina 27858-4354
(919) 816-2202

Admissions Office
CB#7000 MacNider Hall
University of North Carolina at Chapel
Hill
School of Medicine
Chapel Hill, North Carolina 27599-7000
(919) 962-8331

North Dakota

Secretary, Committee on Admissions
University of North Dakota School
of Medicine
501 North Columbia Road
Box 9037
Grand Forks, North Dakota 58202-9037
(701) 777-4221; FAX (701) 777-4942

Ohio

Associate Dean for Admission and
Student Affairs
Case Western Reserve University School
of Medicine
10900 Euclid Avenue
Cleveland, Ohio 44106-4920
(216) 368-3450; FAX (216) 368-4621

Office of Student Affairs/Admissions
University of Cincinnati College
of Medicine
P.O. Box 670552
Cincinnati, Ohio 45267-0552
(513) 558-7314; FAX (513) 558-1165

Admissions Office
Medical College of Ohio
P.O. Box 10008
Toledo, Ohio 43699
(419) 381-4229; FAX (419) 381-4005

Office of Admissions and Educational
Research
Northeastern Ohio Universities
College of Medicine
P.O. Box 95
Rootstown, Ohio 44272-0095
(216) 325-2511

Admissions Committee
270-A Meiling Hall
Ohio State University
College of Medicine
370 West Ninth Avenue
Columbus, Ohio 43210-1238
(614) 292-7137; FAX (614) 292-1544

Office of Student Affairs/Admissions
Wright State University School
of Medicine
P.O. Box 1751
Dayton, Ohio 45401
(513) 873-2934; FAX (513) 873-3322

Oklahoma

Dotty Shaw Killam
University of Oklahoma College
of Medicine
P.O. Box 26901
Oklahoma City, Oklahoma 73190
(405) 271-2331; FAX (405) 271-3032

Oregon

Office of Education and Student Affiars,
L102
Oregon Health Sciences University
3181 S.W. Sam Jackson Park Road
Portland, Oregon 97201
(503) 494-2998; FAX (503) 494-3400

Pennsylvania

Associate Dean for Admissions
Jefferson Medical College of
Thomas Jefferson University
1025 Walnut Street
Philadelphia, Pennsylvania 19107
(215) 955-6983; FAX (215) 923-6939

Admissions Office
Medical College of Pennsylvania and
Hahnemann University School
of Medicine
2900 Queen Lane Avenue
Philadelphia, Pennsylvania 19129
(215) 991-8202; FAX (215) 843-1766

Office of Student Affairs
Pennsylvania State University
College of Medicine
P.O. Box 850
Hershey, Pennsylvania 17033
(717) 531-8755; FAX (717) 531-6225

Director of Admissions and Financial
  Aid
Edward J. Stemmler Hall, Suite 100
University of Pennsylvania School
  of Medicine
Philadelphia, Pennsylvania 19104-6056
(215) 898-8001; FAX (215) 898-0833

Office of Admissions
518 Scaife Hall
University of Pittsburgh School
  of Medicine
Pittsburgh, Pennsylvania 15261
(412) 648-9891; FAX (412) 648-8768

Admissions Office
Suite 305, Student Faculty Center
Temple University School of Medicine
Broad and Ontario Streets
Philadelphia, Pennsylvania 19140
(215) 707-3656; FAX (215) 707-6932

Puerto Rico
Office of Admissions
Universidad Central del Caribe
School of Medicine
Ramon Ruiz Arnau University Hospital
Call Box 60-327
Bayamon, Puerto Rico 00960-6032
(809) 740-1611 Ext. 210;
FAX (809) 269-7550

Admissions Office
Ponce School of Medicine
P.O. Box 7004
Ponce, Puerto Rico 00732
(809) 840-2511; FAX (809) 844-3685

Central Admissions Office
School of Medicine
Medical Sciences Campus
University of Puerto Rico
P.O. Box 365067
San Juan, Puerto Rico 00936-5067
(809) 758-2525, Ext. 5213
FAX (809) 751-3284

Rhode Island
Office of Admissions
Box G-A212
Brown University School of Medicine
Providence, Rhode Island 02912-9706
(401) 863-2149; FAX (401) 863-2660

South Carolina
Office of Enrollment Services
Medical University of South Carolina
171 Ashley Avenue
Charleston, South Carolina 29425
(803) 792-3281; FAX (803) 792-3764

Associate Dean for Student Programs
University of South Carolina School
  of Medicine
Columbia, South Carolina 29208
(803) 733-3325; FAX (803) 733-3328

South Dakota
Office of Student Affairs, Room 105
University of South Dakota School
  of Medicine
414 East Clark Street
Vermillion, South Dakota 57069-2390
(605) 677-5233; FAX (605) 677-5109

Tennessee
Assistant Dean for Admissions and
  Records
East Tennessee State University
James H. Quillen College of Medicine
P.O. Box 70580
Johnson City, Tennessee 37614-0580
(615) 929-6221; FAX (615) 461-7040

Director, Admissions and Records
Meharry Medical College School
  of Medicine
1005 D.B. Todd, Jr. Boulevard
Nashville, Tennessee 37208
(615) 327-6223; FAX (615) 327-6228

University of Tennessee, Memphis
  College of Medicine
800 Madison Avenue
Memphis, Tennessee 38613
(901) 448-5559

Office of Admissions
209 Light Hall
Vanderbilt University School
  of Medicine
Nashville, Tennessee 37232-0685
(615) 322-2145; FAX (615) 343-8397

Texas
Office of Admissions
Baylor College of Medicine
One Baylor Plaza
Houston, Texas 77030
(713) 798-4841

Associate Dean for Student Affairs and
  Admissions
Texas A&M University College
  of Medicine
College Station, Texas 77843-1114
(409) 845-7744; FAX (409) 847-8663

Office of Admissions
Texas Tech University Health Sciences
  Center
School of Medicine
Lubbock, Texas 79430
(806) 743-2297

Office of the Registrar
University of Texas Southwestern
    Medical Center at Dallas
5323 Harry Hines Boulevard
Dallas, Texas 75235-9096
(214) 648-2670; FAX (214) 648-3289

Office of Admissions
G.210, Ashbel Smith Building
University of Texas Medical Branch
    at Galveston
School of Medicine
Galveston, Texas 77555-1317
(409) 772-3517; FAX (409) 772-5753

Office of Admissions
Room G-024
University of Texas Medical School
    at Houston
P.O. Box 20708
Houston, Texas 77225
(713) 792-4711; FAX (713) 794-4238

Medical School Admissions
Registrar's Office
University of Texas Health Science
    Center at San Antonio
7703 Floyd Curl Drive
San Antonio, Texas 78284-7701
(210) 567-2665; FAX (210) 567-2685

Utah
Millie M. Peterson
Director, Medical School Admissions
University of Utah School of Medicine
50 North Medical Drive
Salt Lake City, Utah 84132
(801) 581-7498; FAX (801) 585-3300

Vermont
Admissions Office
E-109 Given Building
University of Vermont College
    of Medicine
Burlington, Vermont 05405
(802) 656-2154

Virginia
Office of Admissions
Eastern Virginia Medical School
700 Olney Road
Norfolk, Virginia 23507-1696
(804) 446-5812; FAX (804) 446-5817

Medical School Admissions
Virginia Commonwealth University
Medical College of Virginia
MCV Station, Box 565
Richmond, Virginia 23298-0565
(804) 828-9629; FAX (804) 828-7628

Medical School Admissions Office,
    Box 235
University of Virginia School
    of Medicine
Charlottesville, Virginia 22908
(804) 924-5571; FAX (804) 982-2586

Washington
Admissions Office (SM-22)
Health Sciences Center T-545
University of Washington
Seattle, Washington 98195
(206) 543-7212

West Virginia
Admissions Office
Marshall University School of Medicine
1542 Spring Valley Drive
Huntington, West Virginia 25755
(304) 696-7312; (800) 544-8514

Office of Admissions and Records
West Virginia University Health
    Sciences Center
P.O. Box 9815
Morgantown, West Virginia 26506
(304) 293-3521; FAX (304) 293-4973

Wisconsin
Office of Admissions and Registrar
Medical College of Wisconsin
8701 Watertown Plank Road
Milwaukee, Wisconsin 53226
(414) 456-8246

Admissions Committee
Medical Sciences Center, Room 1205
University of Wisconsin Medical School
1300 University Avenue
Madison, Wisconsin 53706
(608) 263-4925; FAX (608) 262-2327

Appendix II

· · · · · · · · · ·

CANADIAN
MEDICAL SCHOOLS

Alberta
Admissions Officer
2-45 Medical Sciences Building
University of Alberta
Faculty of Medicine
Edmonton, Alberta
Canada, T6G 2H7
(403) 492-6350; FAX (403) 492-9531

Office of Admissions
University of Calgary
Faculty of Medicine
3330 Hospital Drive, N.W.
Calgary, Alberta
Canada T2N 4N1
(403) 220-6849

British Columbia
Office of the Dean
Faculty of Medicine
Admissions Office
University of British Columbia
317-2194 Health Sciences Mall
Vancouver, British Columbia
Canada V6T 1Z3
(604) 822-4482; FAX (604) 822-6061

Manitoba
Chairman, Admissions Committee
University of Manitoba Faculty
   of Medicine
753 McDermot Avenue
Winnipeg, Manitoba
Canada R3E OW3
(204) 789-3569; FAX (204) 774-8941

Newfoundland
Chairman, Committee on Admissions
Memorial University of Newfoundland
Faculty of Medicine
St. John's, Newfoundland
Canada AlB 3V6
(709) 737-6615; FAX (709) 737-5186

Nova Scotia
Brenda L. Detienne
Admissions Coordinator
Room C-23, Lower Level
Clinical Research Centre
5849 University Avenue
Dalhousie University
Halifax, Nova Scotia
Canada B3H 4H7
(902) 494-1874; FAX (902) 494-3644

Ontario
Admissions and Records
HSC Room lB7-Health Sciences Center
McMaster University
1200 Main Street West
Hamilton, Ontario
Canada L8N 3Z5
(905) 525-9140, extension 22144

Admissions
University of Ottawa Faculty
   of Medicine
451 Smyth Road
Ottawa, Ontario
Canada KlH 8M5
(613) 787-6463; FAX (613) 787-6717

Admissions Office
Queen's University Faculty of Medicine
Kingston, Ontario
Canada K7L 3N6
(613) 545-2542; FAX (613) 545-6884

University of Toronto Faculty
   of Medicine
Toronto, Ontario
Canada M5S lA8
(416) 978-2717; FAX (416) 971-2163

Undergraduate Medical Education
   Office
Medical Sciences Building, Room 100
University of Western Ontario
London, Ontario
Canada N6A SC1
(519) 661-3744; FAX (519) 661-4043

Quebec
Secretary, Admissions Committee
Universite Laval Faculty of Medicine
Ste-Foy, Quebec
Canada GlK 7P4
(418) 646-2492; FAX (418) 656-2733

Admissions Office
McGill University Faculty of Medicine
3655 Drummond Street
Montreal, Quebec
Canada H3G lY6
(514) 398-3517; FAX (514) 398-3595

Committee on Admission
Universite de Montreal Faculty
   of Medicine
P.O. Box 6128, Station Centre-Ville
Montreal, Quebec
Canada H3C 3J7
(514) 343-6265; FAX (514) 343-6629

Admission Office
University of Sherbrooke Faculty
   of Medicine
Sherbrooke, Quebec
Canada JlH 5N4
(819) 564-5208; FAX (819) 564-5378

Saskatchewan
Secretary, Admissions
University of Saskatchewan College
   of Medicine
B103 Health Sciences Building
Saskatoon, Saskatchewan
Canada S7N OWO
(306) 966-8554; FAX (306) 966-6164

INDEX